Wounded Profession

American Medicine
Enters the Age
of Managed Care

Arnold Birenbaum

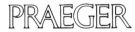
PRAEGER

Westport, Connecticut
London

Library of Congress Cataloging-in-Publication Data

Birenbaum, Arnold.
    Wounded profession : American medicine enters the age of managed care /
Arnold Birenbaum.
        p.   cm.
    Includes bibliographical references and index.
    ISBN 0–275–97389–1 (alk. paper)
    1. Managed care plans (Medical care)—United States.   2. Health maintenance
organizations—United States.   I. Title.
RA413.B54   2002
362.1′04258′0973—dc21   2002066335

British Library Cataloguing in Publication Data is available.

Library of Congress Catalog Card Number: 2002066335
ISBN: 0–275–97389–1

First published in 2002

Praeger Publishers, 88 Post Road West, Westport, CT 06881
An imprint of Greenwood Publishing Group, Inc.
www.praeger.com

Printed in the United States of America

The paper used in this book complies with the
Permanent Paper Standard issued by the National
Information Standards Organization (Z39.48–1984).

10 9 8 7 6 5 4 3 2 1

Dedicated to my grandchildren, Sam and Hannah, who bring joy into my life.

Contents

Preface

This book is about the remaking of the health care system and the consequences of this effort for a major profession. It starts with the rise of medicine in America as a private and largely for-profit clinical practice, aided by the development of the modern academic medical center and financed by a system of indemnity insurance that became increasingly costly to employers, consumers, and government payers. At one time, mainly in the late 1960s and 1970s, medicine was a powerful and highly respected profession in the United States, without parallel. Although still respected, some of its control over its own destiny was lost. It was lost in a struggle with new players in health care—known as managed care organizations—as they came up with new ways of financing and organizing the health care delivery system in the United States.

Financing of health care has always had a strong effect on how the system was organized. Now payment comes with various restrictions on how to conduct medical practice and provide hospital care, calling into question the traditional ways of health care delivery. Managed care, as a way of paying doctors and other providers, is a kind of low-intensity war waged against the culture of private practice, especially specialty providers, and the academic medical centers that depend on patient admissions from their affiliated physicians.

Managed care, through cost shifting to plan participants, is a form of combat also against the indifference to cost displayed by consumers with insurance coverage but with no deductibles and co-payments in their policies. Making members of health care plans aware that visits to the doctor now cost the price of a good lunch, or filling a prescription the cost of a good dinner, reintroduces price sensitivity into consumers' thinking. Putting off a visit now has its rewards, as does settling for a generic drug.

This wholesale effort to rein in costs has led to serious inroads on the way medicine is practiced, how doctors relate to patients, and how much autonomy professionals are permitted in their work. Some of these changes could go beyond saving money, provided that carefully designed studies demonstrate that new clinical practices or health promotion activities produce improvements in health outcomes. There may come a day when breast cancer detection via mammograms is deemed ineffective. And looking further into the future, the promotion of linkages between managed care organizations and public health services, although hardly found today, may also produce better health outcomes via prevention and early intervention.

Despite this potential for improving health care and eliminating unnecessary technology, managed care has been costly to the infrastructure of U.S. health care. The spread of managed care has produced considerable downsizing in the doctors' workshops as hospitals close and academic medical centers are forced to reduce their staffs and close socially valuable programs. The chapters that follow will attempt to document just how much has changed in the course of a decade.

Although managed care has become the dominant form of health care financing and organization today, with only 5 percent of physicians not participating, there is widespread dissatisfaction among doctors with the current state of affairs. Many of those who cannot adapt to the compensation structure or the rules and regulations found in these health plans have taken early retirement. Some doctors, as we will see, have refused to participate in these plans, depending for income on patients willing to pay out of pocket for their services. A few physicians seeking to bond with patients are making house calls or going with their patients to see specialists. In greater numbers, doctors have joined unions at work sites where they are salaried employees and seek collective bargaining rights. Physicians who are independent contractors are also finding collective bargaining attractive.

As I look back on the extraordinary social changes that moved me to write this book on the current state of American medicine during the early stages of the age of managed care, I can't help but think that policy analysis may help the profession regroup in the face of some major challenges. Market forces have led the charge toward the conversion of health insurance from indemnity coverage to cost-driven managed care in its many manifestations. The managed care industry argues forcefully that this is the only way to create affordable health care for all U.S. residents. Perhaps the profession of medicine in the United States will have something to say about how we can have quality care for everyone at a reasonable cost.

Before it can speak in a way that will make the American public listen, the medical profession needs to develop a cadre of leaders who come to the podium as public intellectuals, not just as professionals mainly concerned about their incomes and status. I have attempted to identify the major problems facing the profession as payers for medical care have gained greater power, often at the expense of doctors. Change during the last decade has not been a friend of the medical profession. Yet even the generalizations about managed care that are found in the following pages may not hold forever.

Locally, health care has moved toward high market penetration by managed care plans, but there is no single system of care. Even in maturing markets, where there are few plans available, there is no integration of services or information systems. Nationally, the health care reform debate of the first Clinton administration is likely to make a comeback during our current recession. There is nothing like the loss of employment to focus the mind. Heavy expenses for prescription drugs can work as well on the retired. Some things remain the same the more things change.

SOURCES AND ACKNOWLEDGMENTS

Despite these notes of despair, working on this book has had its pleasures. One of the joys in working in this field is that there are excellent foundations to do policy analyses. I want to acknowledge some of the major contributors to my knowledge and understanding of this field. To write this book I have drawn from a variety of sources, including recent data, sophisticated policy analyses, and systematic health services research. I relied on many articles and editorials from the *New England Journal of Medicine*, the *Journal of the American Medical Association*, and *Health Affairs*. In particular, the continuously fine work of David Blumenthal and John K. Iglehart stands out.

The national press was always there for me because the effect of managed care on the profession of medicine was a story that would not go away. Newspapers that have public policy commitments are often way ahead of the reviewed journals. They were very helpful in dealing with late-breaking policy questions, details on the business end of managed care plans, and how members of the medical profession were responding to change. I am especially indebted to the *New York Times, Washington Post, Wall Street Journal,* and *Boston Globe.* I do wish newspapers that seek to set the national agenda would commit to a health policy page similar to what is found on Wednesdays in the *New York Times* on national and regional educational issues.

Few books have been written on various aspects of how managed care has affected the profession of medicine. Kenneth M. Ludmerer's *Time to Heal: American Medical Education from the Turn of the Century to the Era of Managed Care* was a pleasure to read. Few works in this field have the passion for the subject expressed in this important work on one of America's major institutions—the academic medical center. I learned a great deal from Dr. Ludmerer's historical treatment of the early growth of one of America's treasures, now an endangered institution.

Finally, it's great to acknowledge family help—it is good to know that it is there. My wife, Caroline, was once my in-house editor. Now my son Steven, a writer and a graduate of the LBJ School of Public Affairs, has been exceptionally helpful in editing and criticizing the manuscript. In fact, his suggestions have made this a better book. I remain responsible for all the errors found in this treatise. In no way did the advice of my son even come close to misguiding me.

My son, the policy wonk, has also provided me with some inspiration. His fascination with public intellectuals has opened my eyes to the evident lack of participation in current national debates on health care financing and other issues by members of the medical profession. David Lawrence, retired CEO of Kaiser-Permanente, is an exception to this observation. Even if the good Dr. Lawrence never makes Richard Posner's list of contemporary public intellectuals, he is a wise person who looks to the past, the present, and the future. I hope to follow his lead and do the same, starting with a historical introduction to the study of professions.

An Introduction to the Study
of Professions

If the story of the medical profession in America could be told in three parts, we would be at the beginning of the last section. There was the prelicensing and proprietary medical school era when standards for performance and education were inconsistent. This was followed by the golden age when professional autonomy ruled. The creation of Medicare and Medicaid in 1965, and subsequent efforts to introduce accountability measures for participating hospitals to prevent unnecessary admissions, is often perceived by scholars as the beginning of the end of professional autonomy and control for the profession of medicine. However, the members of the profession did not completely comply with the new rules and regulations, even though their professional societies were supposed to enforce them. Professions have their own power and status in society. They make strenuous efforts to maintain what they have. The power of the medical profession—its capacity to gain a monopoly over the training of its peers and the delivery of services—waxes and wanes over the course of centuries, but never fails to fascinate the discerning eye (Freidson, 1970).

It is no secret that health care practices are common to all societies. Evidence found in the ruins of many early societies demonstrates that sophisticated techniques were used in efforts to help people, relieve suffering, and learn more about injury and illness. Physicians in the southern highlands of Mexico, in the Valley of Oasaca, practiced skull surgery 1,300 years ago. Similar archeological evidence of skull surgery has been found in the ancient civilizations of the Andes Mountains in South America and in Europe as well (Wilkinson, 1975).

Human intervention in matters of illness or injury does not always await the development of a scientific body of verified knowledge. The personal ties among people and the social division of labor promote generalized concern with matters of illness and health. Group life is based on cooperation and interdependence among members to get things done. Thus, the problems presented by illness, disease, and accidents have organizational consequences. Group life is also accompanied by bonds of affection and concern for others, including a sense of being abandoned or let down or feelings of anger when someone cannot live up to previous expectations. In turn, the person who is ill or injured may feel guilty about not being able to perform assigned tasks or angry that others do not show proper concern for his or her absence, suffering, or disability. Disease may be contagious, and societal leaders encourage a variety of measures to counteract it, such as isolation, exile, or magical intervention.

It follows that illness, disease, and accident create social uncertainty that goes beyond individual interests or the interests of a small group such as a family or a work team. Consider the sense of vulnerability created in American society following the terrorist attacks on September 11, 2001. There was, and perhaps still is, a diminution in our sense of security produced by these atrocities.

It is hard to imagine a society that does not make some effort to deal with such unanticipated events. Accordingly, intervention by outside experts on a macrosocial level to interpret these events, even restore our self-confidence, are paralleled by the kind of work that healers do on a microsocial level to explain and make more predictable the future consequences of illness, disease, and accident. Thus, we are better able to deal with the uncertainty produced by these conditions as well as with the physical aspects of the sick person.

Effort, even ineffective effort, can make a difference. Whether physicians and nurses (or witch doctors and herbalists) actually help people get well, or simply see them through the various social and psychological disruptions, they deal with these conditions according to custom. We expect something to be done about current complaints, even when no widely approved treatment exists. Rules are established that dictate who is to perform health activities. In addition, justifications are established to prove that this is the *preferred and best way* to deal with illness, accident, or disease.

Sometimes there is fierce competition between healers following different theories of how the human body works, as in the United States in the nineteenth century. This competition continued in the debate over who should license physicians—states or medical schools. To fully understand the meaning of professions in modern society, it is useful to examine the growth and perhaps the reduction of the power of professions in contemporary society through the powerful lenses of European and American social science.

THE STUDY OF PROFESSIONS IN MODERN SOCIETY

The study of professions in society has a long tradition, although systematic attention to single professions did not take place until the last half of the twentieth century. The nineteenth-century masters of social thought—Marx, Weber, and Durkheim—were sensitive to the ways in which industrialization, economic developments, and modern attitudes were changing relationships between occupational groups, between providers and consumers, and between employers and employees. Marx saw experts doing the bidding of the true wielders of power—captains of the capitalist industrial enterprises that were changing the face of the world. Weber recognized the need to attribute a special status to experts to keep them going in their efforts to make the world more predictable, thereby encouraging the growth of rationality. Durkheim focused on the professional association—the community within the community—as the source of social identity and security in a world characterized by rampant individualism.

As early as 1848, Marx saw the guild system of occupations being destroyed by the dynamics of capitalism. In his brilliant lamentation and futuristic screed, *The Communist Manifesto*, he wrote how "the bourgeoisie has stripped of its halo every occupation hitherto honoured and looked up to with reverent awe." According to Marx and other social analysts of his day, the reduction of independence entailed when a person worked for wages (instead of selling a product or receiving a fee for service) engendered a sense of loss of power and prestige. In turn, the manager and organizer of the labor of others developed a strong sense of mastery, and as Alexis de Tocqueville observed during his travels in America, the development of industry based on mass distribution created a new aristocracy that seemed born to command:

While the workman concentrates his faculties more and more upon the study of a single detail, the master surveys an extensive whole, and the mind of the latter is enlarged in proportion as that of the former is narrowed. In a short time the one will require nothing but physical strength without intelligence; the other stands in need of science, and almost of genius to ensure success. This man resembles more and more the administrator of a vast empire; that man a brute. (Tocqueville, 1945: 169)

Content with pointing out the unintended consequences of democracy and free enterprise, Tocqueville mistook the appearance of narrowness and docility for the complete person. In the nineteenth century, workers often remained convinced that they too could manage and organize industry—sometimes they organized to that end, and sometimes they studied together to improve their minds and become masters of their world. Much of this activity took place away from the workplace and could be hidden from the eyes of even such a formidable observer as Tocqueville.

There is also the need for the scientific knowledge that emerges from this formal and rational organization of the workplace, even more than Tocqueville imagined. The master and workman both become dependent on experts or professionals who can generate knowledge and apply that knowledge. This dependency is based on expectations that the expert provides valuable services. In the case of the physician, cure, prevention, and easing the burden of injury or disease are prized by society. There is also a structure of expectations that approves of members of society seeking help from doctors to solve these kinds of problems.

The medical expert became recognized as an important provider of support services in a society where labor's availability was becoming increasingly important. When production on farms or in factories was based on a goal of selling in a remote marketplace and where transportation was needed for long-distance shipping, efficiency became important. Moreover, breaking down the work process into detailed and specialized labor also meant that later stages in production could not be accomplished unless early tasks were completed. Under these conditions, having the worker away from his or her job, or, for that matter, the entrepreneur away from his or her place of business, was a liability. The division of labor, specialization, and the commercial way of life became recognized as an end in itself (Ure, 1861). By the late eighteenth century, the belief in the rightness of these ways was upheld as a guide to secular behavior. Benjamin Franklin in *Poor Richard's Almanac*, a toolbox for success for those imbued with the spirit of capitalism, wrote that "time is money."

Paradoxically, the more capitalism became a way of life, with its own values of individualism and competition, the more admiration grew for those who gave something back to society. Occupations viewed as involving sacrifice of self-interest for the good of society became increasingly admired. To promote the social benefits believed to come from the services rendered by the profession, either through royal decree as in Europe, or the promotion of voluntary associations as found in the United States, professionals were encouraged to form groups to advance knowledge. In exchange for this involvement in producing knowledge in the service of society, professions were often allowed to monopolize the delivery of a given service, free of the competition of the marketplace. Trust and faith were necessary on the part of the client as the profession increasingly utilized knowledge that the layperson was unable to fully understand.

American sociologists in the first half of the twentieth century, seeking to show that society was real (i.e., external and constraining), and not just made up of billions of interchanges between individuals, found that the study of the professions in modern society was a way of making their case. It was one way of demonstrating how the norms of society could be so powerful, that even when some people had superior knowledge, they would not use it to take advantage of others.

Furthermore, the professional had internalized the profession's code of ethics. For Talcott Parsons (1939), a leading sociological theorist prior to World War II, the rules were introjected to the extent that people complied with the norms of modern society even when not externally constrained to do so. Moreover, professional autonomy was considered a good thing because self-regulation as a form of social control was most compatible with an achievement-oriented society.

Parsons held that the group life of the professions protects against exploitation of the public because all members of the profession internalize an ethical code that restrains them from taking advantage of the buyer. These scruples are supposed to keep professionals from acting unfairly toward clients; they are also a foundation for making independent judgments in assessing clients, not merely coming up with convenient reviews. If the Arthur Andersen firm had done a truly independent audit of Enron, it would have called into question this high-flying client's unusual business practices long before the Texas-based energy trading company crashed and burned.

Control over the behavior of members of the profession is seen, according to this theory, to be best established through self-regulation, not through outside intervention. Peer review, another name for self-regulation, becomes the measure of all meaningful things in the profession because of the specialized quality of the work performed. And this work is considered vital: Society has a compelling interest in seeing that it gets done, for individuals need to be cared for in order to feel part of society as well as to carry out or return to their full-time obligations.

Some observers, even before Parsons, were skeptical of the extent to which professions were protective of the public. George Bernard Shaw, the Anglo-Irish playwright, viewed a profession as a conspiracy against the laity. Regardless of Parsons's correctness, it would be useful to examine how a profession gained the capacity for monopoly over a task vital to society. How did the profession of medicine convince society at large, and particularly elite groups, that they should be the sole providers of these services?

Whether the functions professionals perform in a generic sense are concrete or symbolic, and whatever the cause for recognizing their special authority—one based on society's innate wisdom in opting for autonomy for this unique work community or one that identifies a successful marketing of a service—the outcome has been the same. A few major professions—namely law, medicine, and engineering—have gained control over their work environments and the requirements for entry into the profession; they have established techniques for categorizing the problematic aspects of daily life and set up routine procedures for dealing with them. That experts have achieved this recognition or stature in society may be partly a result of the knowledge base of the profession and partly a result of the justifications created to encourage people to attribute to them dominance over certain vital services (Freidson, 1970). Furthermore, Parsons's approach, which became known as the functionalist school of sociology, saw technical and professional recognition as the outcome of scientific progress resulting from autonomy for the professional community. He did not examine whether professions sought to stifle competition and gain advantages. He certainly never anticipated that a profession such as medicine could lose some of its power in modern society.

In 1970, Eliot Freidson's work on the application of knowledge and professional dominance suggested a more interactive and interpretive path toward professional autonomy. Like many other forms of social mobility, professional autonomy was also a path to power and status. Starting with the assumptions that all occupations seek to control entry into them and have strong preferences as to the actual work environment where services are rendered, he was able to call into question the idea that the value of medicine, or any other profession, to society was self-evident. In a carefully constructed argument, largely based on historical material, this sociologist of the professions proved that medicine received autonomy *prior* to demonstrating technical effectiveness. Clearly, medicine made an effort to convince society that it should be self-regulating. The quest for autonomy and dominance is part of all campaigns for professionalization.

On another level, Freidson was able to demonstrate that medicine was perceived as a healing art even when proven therapies were of no value to patients. In medical practice, he concluded, doctors were trained to find disease, and sometimes they found it when it was not there because the institutionalized norms pushed them in that direction, making the sin of overlooking disease more serious than identifying it when it was not really there. Moreover, the very act of being treated, even with placebos, was shown to make people feel better.

Freidson was able to take apart Parsons's theory of the professions because Freidson was more widely read on the history of medicine, understood more about how impressions of success were created, even in the professions, and found support from other sociologists who specialized in the study of the professions. This powerful argument against the teleologic elements in functional analysis was supported by scholarly work on the legal profession, which showed that lawyers gained autonomy without a scientific body of knowledge (Rueschemeyer, 1964). The linkage to state legislatures seemed especially warm and cozy to observers of the legal profession.

Evidence from other sources suggested that medicine's quest for a monopoly over health services came about at the right time from a public health perspective. The elimination of famine from some parts of the world, mainly where industrialization advanced most rapidly in the nineteenth century, made people more capable of withstanding infection (McKeown, 1965). Medicine became more effective as a service when it had access to this secret ally—good nutrition. Improvements in sanitation in the late nineteenth century via the development of enclosed sewer systems and the purification of the water supply also reduced the likelihood of infection from waterborne diseases, such as cholera. Personal hygiene improved in the early twentieth century as public health authorities urged people to wash their hands after using the toilet. And so ironically, treatment became the central foci of health care, even when preventive measures made it possible for the medical profession to take the spotlight in the quest for licensing.

The theme of the need to gain governmental support for efforts to professionalize a craft was echoed across the Atlantic. Around the same time that Freidson's work on the profession of medicine was published, a British sociologist, Terrance Johnson (1972), began to outline a methodology for the study of professions that focused on their relationship with those powerful credentialing bodies—national and state governments. Insofar as any government institution by law can grant a shelter from market competition, then they ought to be closely scrutinized to understand how one occupation gets sheltered and another does not. The granting or the removing of a professional monopoly on specific tasks is a key event in the history of a profession. Consequently, Johnson suggested that the acquisition of power and status become a sequence of events that can be broken down and studied historically and comparatively, instead of focusing on the supposed generic elements of a professional versus a nonprofessional occupation.

Although Johnson sometimes suggested that some occupations are more likely to become professions than others because of the extensive degree of uncertainty in the work that is performed, he refocused on credentialing. In a rare aphorism by a sociologist, Johnson observed that "a profession is not, then an occupation, but a means of controlling an occupation" (p. 45). The means of controlling a professionalized occupation is through credentials. This is a method of control based on standardization of the performer's education.

By establishing uniform educational requirements as a condition of entry into practice, the profession creates an entry barrier that sharply improves the market situation for existing practitioners. In a later opus, *Professional Powers* (1986), Freidson proffered the idea that credentialing serves to create "an occupational cartel which gains and preserves monopolistic control over the supply of a good or service in order to enhance the income of its members by protecting them from competition by others" (p. 63). Max Weber would have found this definition compatible with his conceptualization of the guild system of production during precapitalist epochs. The difference between the professional association and the guild is that the professional association does not deliberately restrict production of services, only the production of producers. The profession also controls the university-based educational programs that turn out newly minted professionals.

Professions are, then, unique occupations that have gained exclusivity in solving other people's problems. However, they do so at a cost: using labor-market shelters built around the higher educational credentials to gain some marginal power and a good deal of social status (Freidson, 1986: 109). Thus their advice cannot be easily ignored because it is bought at a high price, even when the technology used has not always proven to be effective. In sum, a profession many gain autonomy and control but it may not last forever. The current form of control over health care delivery exercised by the profession of medicine is challenged by those who pay for health care and those who receive it.

REFERENCES

Freidson, E. 1970. *The Profession of Medicine*. New York: Dodd, Mead.
Freidson, E. 1986. *Professional Powers*. Chicago: University of Chicago Press.
Johnson, T. 1972. *Professions and Power*. London: MacMillan.
McKeown, T. 1965. *The Modern Rise of Population*. New York: Academic Press.
Parsons, T. 1939. *Essays in Sociology*. Glencoe, IL: The Free Press.
Rueschemeyer, D. 1964. "Doctors and lawyers: A comment on the theory of the professions." *The Canadian Review of Sociology and Anthropology 1*: 17–30.
Tocqueville, A. de. 1945. *Democracy in America* (Vol. 2). Trans. Henry Reeve. New York: Vintage Books.
Ure, A. 1861. *The Philosophy of Manufactures*. London: H.G. Bohn.
Wilkinson, R.G. 1975. "Techniques of ancient skull surgery." *Natural History* (October): 94–101.

1

Health Care on the National Agenda

The clash between managed care and the medical profession needs to be seen not only in the context of the story of the profession of medicine in the United States, but also in the context of efforts to reform health care and the changes that followed its failure. The medical profession is not wholly without blame in the most serious effort to reform health care since the advent of Medicare and Medicaid.

After a decade of exhaustive debate and incremental tinkering with the health care system, the issues of quality of care, cost, and access remain on the national agenda. Our gentle and prosperous entry into the twenty-first century has not seen a resolution to these major problems in the American health care system. The displacements and disruptions caused by managed care are not responsible for all unresolved problems. Still, managed care is identified as a culprit. The prosperity of the 1990s allowed for employers to submit to employee demands that health care plans supply a choice of providers and the elimination of the functioning of primary care providers as "gatekeepers" to the specialists in the plan. Concern about choice was based on a commonsense view that consumers should not be subject to bureaucratic runarounds to save money for their employer, the purchaser of the coverage, or the managed care plan itself.

Although the 1960s and 1970s brought out some compelling arguments that "less is more," this countercultural aphorism does not sit well with the health care buying public today. There was a backlash against rationing of care. The identification of the practice of stinting on services became part of the lexicon of health policy analysis in the 1990s. Patients began to question doctors when they said that the best course of treatment was no treatment, despite the clear evidence from numerous studies that refraining from intervening was sometimes wise, or that the unwanted consequences of surgery or other invasive treatments might be worse than living with a disease. The insured public sought to do away with doctors saying no to them when it came to getting care.

We have now come full circle. There is public and professional concern that managed care plans hold back on services. Consequently, these unwanted policies and practices prevent patients from recovering quickly, diminish the quality of their lives, or even create risks to life. Concern about stinting helped promote congressional action. A patients' bill of rights with some real penalties for limiting access to services was tantalizingly close to passage in Congress at the beginning of the new century. Naturally, the American Association of Health Plans (AAHP), the trade association for the managed care industry, strongly opposed passage of the Norwood/Dingle legislation. So, too, did President George W. Bush, who feared that the trial lawyers of America would make out like bandits if patients had the right to sue managed care plans in state courts. Even in his home state of Texas, the patients' bill of rights that passed into law without his signature when he was governor did not convince the president that protections were needed in the courts.

Nor would this occupant of the White House find it necessary to take government action to rein in the costs of prescription drugs. A plethora of new and very expensive medications save lives, extend life in the face of cancer, congestive heart disease, and AIDS, to name but three major killers, or make living more satisfying and productive by limiting symptoms, as in the case of arthritis. Now, the national agenda includes concern about elderly people on fixed incomes and with no prescription insurance plan, as well as others who depend on expensive medications to survive. Many Americans complain about, and are burdened by, their high out-of-pocket costs. The remedies found in the prescription-policy positions issued by George W. Bush and Al Gore in the endless 2000 presidential race took radically different approaches, and this was also true of other health care issues.

After hearing the candidates debate, reading their statements on health care in the October 19, 2000, issue of the *New England Journal of Medicine*, and, of course, seeing the results of the congressional election, I inferred that there is no secure middle ground on which to build a bipartisan consensus necessary to pass significant legislation to create universal health care access. Presidential support for the Norwood/Dingle bill does not exist. There is sufficient support for this bill in the Senate. However, President Bush is seeking to reduce the capacity of patients to sue their health plan in any legislation he would support.

Perhaps even more significant, consumer advocates and health care policy analysts alike point to the growing number of Americans without insurance. Can this be in a modern industrial and affluent society? There are 42.6 million uninsured Americans who have limited access to care. And this was at the end of the longest period of sustained economic growth in American history!

Still, hope was alive that some more people in the United States without insurance would gain coverage. In late November of 2000, three old enemies agreed that more Americans should be insured. A proposal made by an odd coalition of players in the health care field—the Health Insurance Association of America (HIAA), the American Hospital Association (AHA), and the consumer advocacy organization Families USA—called for extending Medicaid, the federal-state medical assistance program for the poor; making adults eligible through the Children's Health Insurance Program; and offering tax credits for corporations that employ low-wage workers (Pear, 2000). It is an astonishing partnership. As the representative of sellers of indemnity insurance, the HIAA was a major roadblock to the Clinton Health Plan in 1993 and 1994, and the AHA and Families USA were supporters of universal coverage features of what was known then as the Health Security Act. Are the Harry and Louise commercials, the devastating brainchild of the HIAA, finally in full retirement? I don't think so. They may come back in new guises.

The budget deficits generated by the repairs after the attacks in New York and Washington, D.C., plus the cost of the war on terrorism in Afghanistan, may not make extending health care coverage to more Americans an issue high on the national agenda. A pragmatic approach is required in any event. The gap between the insured and the uninsured is as large as the gap between social classes in the United States. Commentators talk about the failure of providers and consumers to communicate. There is no doubt that communication between providers and patients can be improved. The irony is that some Americans would be pleased to communicate in any way possible: They may not have the financial capacity or private or public insurance to become depersonalized. Mostly invisible because they are politically weak, the uninsured simply live on the margins of the health-care delivery system.

This does not mean that there has been no change, and that no further change will take place, in the organization and financing of American health care. At what is almost 14 percent of the gross domestic product, a measure of all the goods and services produced inside the United States, and still growing, with an estimate that it will increase to 16.2 percent in 2008, health care is too important to both elected officials and business leaders, not to mention the general population, to leave alone (Blumenthal, 2001).

Purchasers—including employers, the congressional stewards of Medicare and Medicaid, and consumers—have been insisting since the early 1980s that health care has become unaffordable. The effort to do something about the high cost set in motion enormous changes in how the financial risks of providing care are to be shared between payers, providers, and patients. The consequences have been enormous. Physicians, in negotiation with managed care plans, now offer deep discounts to payers so that their usual and customary fees were merely talking points and not serious charges for any payers. When payers control access to patients, or as they say in the insurance business, "covered lives," physicians see the value of joining the networks that generate revenues. They may hold their noses, as my dear wife would say, but they join up. Perhaps veteran doctors saw longtime patients leave their practices when their employers contracted with managed care organizations; their Medicare patients also signed up for health maintenance organizations (HMOs) in large numbers in the early 1990s. And young doctors with medical school debt, mortgages, and children to educate, in recognition of the new economics of medicine, are well aware of what they have to do to maintain sufficient income to cover their expenses and lead comfortable lives. Market reform has eclipsed public policy reform.

Consider how this has affected medical careers. A new physician appears to be emerging. Significantly, by the year 2000, some medical students who wanted to be well-paid physicians were in dual-degree programs. These programs did not combine traditional alliances such as cell biology and medicine. These stalwarts were pioneers: By signing up for a six-year program, they would receive a medical degree and a master's in business administration (MBA) (Ellis, 2000). Sustained by the bright and shiny optimism of the American business culture, even doctors who have been in practice for many years are seeking MBAs as a way of adapting to the new competitive environment. Some physicians have fought back by organizing and forming their own managed care plans. Managed care plans in some regions have bought up physician practices and made the doctors salaried employees, thereby eliminating some of the competition. Other physicians have sought early retirement rather than have to deal with the rules and regulations of managed care plans. And still others have found asylum, and lower incomes, in an academic career, focusing on the study of medical ethics or the changing organization and delivery of health-care services and medical practices.

To fully understand the dynamics that produced the managed care revolution, let's return to the 1980s and review how the payers significantly took charge of health care and consequently muted professional sovereignty in the marketplace and autonomy in their workshop—the acute care hospital. Although there may have been earlier indications of capitalists-as-payers discomfort in the United States with rising costs, as forcefully argued by Eliot Krause (1996), the critical mass for across-the-board change did not emerge until a Democratic Congress and a Republican president (Ronald Reagan) produced legislation to allow for prospective payment by Medicare for hospital stays. It is noteworthy that sociologists George Ritzer and David Walczak (1986) were conceptualizing these changes in the public payment system as part of a process that would deprofessionalize physicians. Without trying to introduce purple prose, I would say that these changes were harbingers of a fateful future.

Efforts to rein in costs in Medicare were inevitable. The last New Deal legislation of the Roosevelt era was part of President Lyndon Baines Johnson's Great Society. A very liberal Congress was willing to ride his coattails in 1964 and subsequently supported his Medicare and Medicaid legislation. It wasn't long before reality set in as lawmakers learned that the country had to pay for the war in Vietnam and social legislation at the same time. Legislators were shocked by the rise in the cost of the Medicare program after its initiation in 1965. Consequently, earlier Congresses tried to make doctors more accountable for their decisions. It was not just a matter of cost. Concern about quality was also an issue. Within the medical profession, voluntary efforts to protect patients were introduced by the American College of Surgeons in its reformist days, as early as 1913. Legislation in the form of amendments to the Social Security Act (P.L. 92-603) was passed in 1972 and called for hospitals receiving Medicare funds to set up utilization review committees, a form of quality assurance to prevent inappropriate hospital admissions, so they could do self-regulation. These requirements went beyond the establishment of standing committees, wherein periodic mortality and morbidity inquiries were held, and ongoing medical record review, efforts to make doctors accountable to their peers. Hospitals had to have these programs in place to be certified by the Joint Commission on the Accreditation of Hospitals (JCAH). Now called the Joint Commission on the Accreditation of Health Organizations (JCAHO), this national organization was established in 1952 by the hospital industry to generate uniformity in its caregiving member organizations.

Additional and more effective pressure to control physician decision making came from a need for hospitals to avoid litigation and the increasing costs of institutional malpractice insurance. In the 1965 landmark Darling Case, hospitals themselves became legally liable for their medical staff's clinical performance, including those doctors with admitting privileges. Now financially accountable and responsible as corporations, hospitals became concerned about the quality of medical decision making and health care delivery that occurred in their environs.

Federal legislation assigned responsibilities to county and state medical societies to make sure hospital admissions were medically necessary and met professional standards. Professional associations were also asked to consider whether the needed services could be provided more economically in an alternative way. In addition, information was to be collected on physicians and patients to establish regional standards of care. Physicians and hospitals found to be abusing these norms could be censured by the local professional society and removed from participation in the Medicare program.

Designated as professional standard review organizations (PSROs), overseeing bodies were established to prevent the delivery of unnecessary services that would have to be paid for by Medicare. They were responsible for reviewing the local hospital's own utilization review programs to make sure these institutions were making a good-faith effort. Hospital administrators were now responsible not only for the delivery of services but also for collecting and providing information on the process and outcome of care. Quality of patient care was placed clearly in the hands of hospital managers, not only medical staff, and the audits that they had to carry out to assure quality were also to be used to change practices and performances. These programs, along with various evolutions of the standards set by the JCAHO, were designed to promote quality and save money at the same time.

HOSPITAL UTILIZATION REVIEW, COST-CONTROL EFFORTS, AND PHYSICIAN AUTONOMY

The investigation of the overutilization of services almost always finds that a minority of doctors or patients account for a disproportionate share of costs. The research undertaken to reduce inappropriate hospitalization and average length of stay reflects the view that medicine is made up of physicians predisposed to hospitalize and patients who are more likely to be hospitalized. Older physicians are more likely to hospitalize patients inappropriately than younger physicians, and women were more likely to be hospitalized unnecessarily than men (Siu, Manning, and Benjamin, 1990). Wickizer (1990: 343), in a comprehensive review of the literature on the effect of utilization review on hospital use and expenditures, found that "PSROs reduced hospital use through their admission review activity rather than through their continued stay review." The presence of utilization review authorities may discourage physicians from even trying to hospitalize patients where they could be treated as outpatients. Few sanctions were ever directed toward delinquent doctors who misused scarce resources. The profession closed ranks to protect its public reputation. A cynic might regard this new form of accountability as putting the fox in charge of the henhouse.

In fact, federal laws and regulations prevented hospitals and state peer review organizations from releasing information to patients or their relatives about whether the care they received met professionally acceptable standards, without the physician's permission. As I write, a new initiative by the Department of Health and Human Services would change its policies to allow Medicare beneficiaries upon request to obtain information about substandard care (Pear, 2001: A1, A12).

Tens of thousands of Medicare patients file complaints each year about the quality of the care they receive from doctors and hospitals. But in many cases, patients get no useful information because doctors can block the release of assessments of their performance. (Pear, 2001: A1)

Although the outgoing Clinton administration appointees changed the rules before inauguration day for George W. Bush, it remains uncertain whether the new administration will accept this change. An administration unfriendly to trial lawyers and malpractice suits may not take kindly to this effort to increase access to information about failed medical work.

There are also medical concerns about raising the bar too high to admit patients to the hospital with relatively unserious symptoms. Many health policy experts applaud efforts to prevent unnecessary hospitalization and prolonged stays, but some of the criteria used may not be cost-effective because lags in admissions can mean a longer hospital stay from having to treat a sicker person. Not all efforts to reduce hospitalization have benign outcomes. Because it takes longer to get to the surgeon today with managed care programs and it is more difficult to gain permission to perform surgery where positive signs of appendicitis are not always present, patients are more likely to have a marked increase in sickness or morbidity when the appendectomy is actually performed (Cacioppo et al., 1989).

Admissions, even unnecessary admissions, up until the mid-1980s, helped the hospital survive financially. Long stays helped sustain income as well. Hospitals were paid a fixed rate per day, plus an additional percentage to cover administrative costs, based on what was known as a "cost plus" formula. The introduction of the prospective-payment system (PPS) and various cost-control mechanisms now used by most third-party payers (Relman, 1991: 854) had a deep impact on hospital financing and the autonomy of physicians. PPS was a monumental change in the way hospitals were supported financially, and its introduction marked the end of what Bruce Vladeck (1990), the former director of Medicare, called the gravy years for all hospitals. It also disciplined the medical workforce in new ways.

A PROSPECTIVE-PAYMENT SYSTEM

By the early 1980s, Congress had given up on the idea that self-regulation would work to contain hospital costs, and introduced a program to alter the way hospitals were paid for patient care by the agency responsible for running Medicare—the Health Care Financing Administration (HCFA). In the year 2001, HCFA morphed into the Center for Medicare and Medicaid Services (CMS). In the past, cost control in hospital expenditures specifically and health care in general, after the initiation of Medicare and Medicaid, occurred only in the 1970s when several states adopted all-payer systems to regulate hospital rates and when the Nixon administration's Economic Stabilization Program between 1972 and 1974 froze wages and prices for all industries (Schroeder and Cantor, 1991: 1100). Now it was time to keep the entire financing system of Medicare afloat.

Congress was warned in the early 1980s by the stewards of the social security system that the money for the Hospital Insurance Trust Fund, designated Medicare Part A, the payer of hospital bills, would be depleted before the beginning of the next decade if cost control was not introduced. After first freezing payments to hospitals for a three-year period, Congress devised a payment reform plan, and made it law in 1982, to reimburse hospitals according to a formula that was set up in advance of each hospital stay. Referred to as a prospective-payment system, its goals were to control costs, make hospitals more efficient users of resources, and maintain the quality of care.

How were these goals to be accomplished? A new way of paying required a strong intellectual justification for giving up the cost-plus arrangements then in place. A provocative idea was already on the shelf in the halls of academe. Originally developed as a tool to measure variability in length of stay by John Thompson, a Yale School of Management and Organization professor, the rationale for changing the financial incentives was based on the idea that good care was independent of time spent in the hospital.

The first two goals would be met by the establishment and use of the diagnosis-related groups (DRGs), a complex system of classification of patients by 470 disease categories related to organ systems of the body. These identities would be assigned to patients at admission, regardless of the differences in the seriousness of the illness from the patient's and hospital's perspective. It is possible that some patients might require more direct care in hospital than others, even with the same disease. For each condition, such as simple pneumonia, the hospital would receive a flat rate of predetermined payment. These rates were based on the collection and organization of data on the length-of-stay averages by disease for the entire country before the introduction of the DRG system as the method of payment. Adjustments also were made in the rates of payment to take into account that teaching hospitals had additional costs.

Under this prospective-payment scheme, hospitals were considered to be in a position to strike a balance between patients, making money on some and losing on others. This kind of reasoning would make sense if each hospital had a proportionate share of the difficult and the "cream puff" cases. Yet it was observed that some hospitals disproportionately cared for more of the population with a greater level of sickness (for example, the poor) than other hospitals.

Some other problems can be predicted by the structure of rewards and incentives built into this new effort at cost control. It was also the goal of the creators of the prospective-payment system to make hospitals more aware of costs and therefore more efficient in delivery of inpatient services. Getting patients out faster, even when it might result in the loss of some appropriate in-hospital care for some patients, would become a prime consideration in determining whether to extend the use of DRGs to other payers.

In this respect, acute-care hospitals were constrained to do less testing for patients, since they were no longer reimbursed by Medicare for each test performed; to look for easy cases rather than difficult ones; and to become more proficient through specialization in the performance of certain inpatient treatments (such as open-heart surgery). In addition, the DRG-based payment system made hospitals more market-oriented as they sought out new admissions to keep their beds filled.

Congress attempted to maintain the high quality of hospital care despite the introduction of incentives to discharge patients early by reformulating the PSRO system as a monitor. Created in 1982, the peer review organizations (PROs) formed a new system that used physician-based organizations, which were explicitly forbidden from delegating review functions to hospitals. Moreover, PROs were to be proactive in getting physicians to change their practice behavior. Contracts with PROS were based upon giving these monitoring agencies the task of achieving such objectives as reducing the rate of overall admissions or the percentage of inappropriate admissions. Contracts were written in such a way that outcomes were specified in numerical reductions in the use of resources (Weitzman, 1990: 375).

The reformation of the peer review system hardly is reassuring to Medicare patients. The previously mentioned concerns suggest that the average length of stay could become the providers' upper limit on stays—that patients might not be getting enough care after the introduction of the prospective-payment system. Might not hospitals become less willing to give good care if they were not appropriately compensated? What were the clinical effects of introducing the DRG system of payment to hospitals? Were patients not being discharged quicker and sicker?

To answer these questions the Health Care Financing Administration funded an elaborate study to examine the effects of the DRG-based prospective-payment system on the quality of care of hospitalized Medicare patients. Conducted by the health program of the Rand Corporation, a West Coast think tank and research company, a pre- and post-DRG study contrasted data on 16,758 Medicare patients who were hospitalized in one of five states prior to and subsequent to 1983. Concentrating half their sample in 1981–82, and the other half in 1985–86, the investigators attempted to control for patient sickness upon admission because adverse outcomes such as mortality could be because they were patients near death rather than because of poor-quality care (Kahn et al., 1990). The investigators found no increase in mortality during the 180 days after hospitalization for the group hospitalized under the prospective-payment system. In addition, the adequacy of care was also supported by the lack of any increase in readmissions for the post-DRG group. Finally, there was no indication that nursing homes were being overwhelmed by admissions or prolonged stays under the new payment system. The process and outcome analysis did uncover one disquieting finding: The prospective-payment system significantly increased the likelihood that a patient would be discharged in an unstable condition (Rogers et al., 1990: 1989). However, remember that the mortality rate and readmission rate did not increase.

The idea of physician accountability caught on. If we fast-forward to the last decade, a substantial percentage of clinicians were subject to review by their managed care plans. Remler et al. (1997) reported that in a 1995 survey of physicians in clinical practice, 59 percent said their patients were reviewed for length of stay, 45 percent for site of care, and 39 percent for how well the treatment fit the disease.

The paradoxical effect of prospective payment is also suggested by these findings. It is possible that doctors, nurses, and other staff in hospitals may act more carefully and deliberately in their work now that their patients' time in the hospital bed is limited. More thinking and communicating may occur under the constraints of the DRG system than occurred before. There were some benefits to the system of effective pressure. Most important, doctors were subject to a new discipline that restricted their professional autonomy. Physicians who could not work under this new regime would lose their admitting privileges at hospitals dependent on Medicare revenues. A doctor without hospital affiliation would not be able to provide continuous care for a patient when the patient most needed it. Other pressures on hospitals and physicians came from the business sector.

AMERICAN BUSINESS LEADERS SEEK TO REIN IN THE
COST OF EMPLOYEE HEALTH BENEFITS

The medical profession was under the gun in the 1980s, but it was not the only elite group in trouble. The country started the Reagan years in a deep recession that ended the stagflation of the late 1970s, a combination of high prices, soaring interest rates, and stubborn unemployment rates. As mentioned previously, the stewards of the social security system were angry about rising hospital costs. Costs were of even more immediate concern to private-sector payers. Business leaders in that decade addressed the general problem of paying for health-care benefits for their employees. An aging population, with many retirees and a mature workforce, led business leaders to seek government-sponsored solutions in a land that relies on market solutions to social problems. Profit-driven CEOs and chairmen of the board in our most respected blue-chip corporations were willing to consider national insurance programs to remove the burden of health-care costs from their ledgers. They were also open to considering new forms of coverage for employees during a decade when costs rose by as much as 17 percent from one year to the next (Freudenheim, 1991: D1). Even a reduction in the increase, let's say from 17 to 10 percent, began to look good to those business leaders involved in heated head-to-head competition with foreign companies for market share here and abroad.

American business moguls who competed with international companies that sold similar commodities sought to cut their production costs. They often complained that employee health care benefits on a per car basis cost more than the steel that went into producing the vehicle. Comparisons on 1983 Japanese and American labor costs in the automobile industry found comparable wage rates, but the fringe-benefit packages made American labor costs expensive: On an hourly basis, American total labor costs were 60 percent higher (Thurow, 1984: 1569). Economists pointed out almost a decade ago that Japanese plant investment, double that of American industry, helped to account for greater labor productivity. Modernization for the American auto industry was held back by added financial burdens of health-care benefits. Cash reserves that once were used to secure loans went to pay for health care for aging workers or retired employees.

Data presented in the 1989 *Health Care Financing Review* (Levit, Freeland, and Waldo, 1989), a Social Security Administration publication, comparing the annual growth in payments for health benefits by corporations as a share of pretax profits, pointed to similar conclusions. Health costs in 1965 were 8.7 percent of pretax profits, whereas in 1987 they were 48.6 percent. Something had to be done. Health policy analysts started to identify the problem as related to the way patients were insured and doctors were compensated for care.

Health benefits, whether through government or corporate financing, have become increasing costly in American society. When a third party pays for the service, consumers sometimes seek care when it is not medically necessary. Moreover, some health-policy analysts describe providers as the real consumers of care, since, as decision makers, they sometimes order unneeded tests or make questionable referrals. These unnecessary visits and other services may not be done deliberately to run up the costs, but the ultimate payers were not happy.

Self-restraint is hard to manage when we know the services we seek are going to be paid for. The logic is that if something is paid for, it will be provided, even when it is marginally useful to the patient. Patients and providers act as if in collusion, giving the ultimate payers—employers, social security payroll tax contributors, or general taxpayers—little chance for containing costs.

Lester Thurow (1984: 1570) captures the self-perpetuating and expansive nature of such an interlocked system of incentives to spend and use, use and spend.

In these circumstances an insurance system ends up having no constraints. Insurance companies have an interest in higher health-care expenditures, since higher expenditures leads to higher corporate incomes. Doctors practicing in the fee-for-service system have a personal interest in prescribing services, since they raise their own income by doing so, and in an insurance system doctors know that they will not be directly raising costs for their patients if they do so. With insurance, patients have no interest in restraining their own health-care expenditures. The result, not surprisingly, is a system with exploding expenditures.

In the 1980s, a good number of American business leaders, such as Lee Iacocca, former chairman of the Chrysler Corporation, began to take a startling unbusinesslike position in favor of national health insurance. They concluded that our segmented payment system was working against them. Cost shifting meant that corporations were paying a disproportionate share of health-care costs. Since controls on costs were introduced in Medicare and Medicaid, the way the very poor in the United States get medical assistance, they found increases in prices for services for those covered by private insurance. All-payer legislation in many states permitted hospitals and academic medical centers to levy a surcharge on insured patients who were hospitalized to make up the shortfall for publicly insured patients and those who received uncompensated care.

More significant, employers were beginning to seek new ways of reducing the costs of health benefits for employees through shifting more of the financial responsibility to workers. Benefits officers sought financial and practical solutions to their companies' rising costs for health care coverage. In addition, insurers introduced various forms of managed care as alternatives to indemnity insurance and traditional third-party payment. In the former case, employees paid a greater percentage of the premiums for health insurance and also assumed larger co-payments when they made a visit to the doctor. In the latter solution, insurers began to organize managed care plans with networks of providers in ways designed to drive down utilization, making for fewer visits to doctors, and compel providers to assume some of the financial risks for their treatment decisions. Additionally, managed care plans sought and received discounts from participating physicians and hospitals for sending their covered patients to them. Members of a proud and sovereign occupation were hardly holding out for their right to set "customary, prevailing, and reasonable" fees as they did when Medicare was introduced in the enabling legislation of President Lyndon Baines Johnson. Wilbur Cohen, the architect of Medicare and Medicaid, knew that being generous to physicians would lead to the development of an expensive system. But in the 1960s, physician organizations such as the American Medical Association (AMA) were strongly opposed to doctors being paid by the government. They were afraid that it was the first step toward nationalization of all health care and that, ultimately, physicians would be employees rather than operating their practices as independent businesses. Early HMOs, such as Kaiser-Permanente on the West Coast and the Health Insurance Program started in New York City, were despised by physicians in private practice. They said that any doctor who worked for a salary was an inferior or incompetent practitioner. Times have changed, as physicians seeking patients, from whatever source, made managed care more attractive to the medical world. These are enormous changes as the last century ended, especially for members of a proud profession.

THE DOCTOR GLUT

Why did doctors and hospitals agree to reduce their fees and abide by the rules invoked by managed care plans? A growing oversupply of physicians and hospital beds made joining managed care plans a necessity. Since the subject of this treatise is the effect of managed care on the profession of medicine, I will concentrate on data that show why physicians were willing to join plans, despite the profession's organizational, and physicians' largely personal, allegiance to fee-for-service medicine and indemnity insurance.

Forty years ago, medical and health planners, and some ordinary citizens as well, were concerned about the shortage of physicians in the

United States. In 1960 there were only 140 physicians for every 100,000 people, and there was enormous regional variability in the distribution of these medical and osteopathic doctors. By 1970, the situation had only slightly improved. There were 156 physicians for the same 100,000 Americans, hardly an enormous increase during a remarkable decade that saw the initiation of Medicare and Medicaid (National Center for Health Statistics, 1985: 106). These programs radically expanded the market for medical care in the United States. Congress initially passed the Health Professions Educational Assistance Act in 1963, and later extended the benefits to medical schools in 1976, to deal with the perceived physician shortage (Feldstein, 1986).

Several new medical schools were started in the 1970s, creating a total of 125 for the country (the same number there are today). In addition, the number of osteopathic medical schools increased from fourteen to nineteen. The number of graduates of schools of osteopathy, which essentially produce primary care physicians who work in areas where medical doctors are in short supply, almost doubled when figures are compared from 1980 and 1997 (Howell, 1999: 1467).

Moreover, the physician shortage was particularly devastating in the area of primary care since most medical students were deciding to become specialists. General practice was being relegated to the scrap heap along with the house call and the direct payment to the doctor for services rendered. Critics began to recognize a strange paradox in American health care: We utilized technologically advanced medicine to deal with serious threats to life or functioning, but it was hard to find doctors to do day-to-day prevention, health promotion, and even treatment of minor (and even serious) maladies. Managed care plans, by creating incentives, accelerated the shift to a health-care system built around the primary care provider.

Congress appropriated funds to assist medical schools to expand their capacity to educate more doctors. Health policy planners created advance practice nursing and the physician assistant as ways of improving access to primary care without using overtrained physicians to do these tasks. The physician shortage of the 1960s and 1970s that fueled the physician extender movement (e.g., nurse practitioners and physician's assistants) and led to the increased class size of medical schools, quickly gave way to the surplus of physicians found today, with a record 220 physicians for every 100,000 people in the population (Roback, Randolph, and Seidman, 1993).

As more Americans began to sign up with managed care plans and HMOs, the calculation of how many physicians were needed per 100,000 people in the population was sharply below the figures established for the early 1990s. Estimates from that same period suggested that somewhere between 120 and 138 physicians were needed for every 100,000 people. And the distribution between primary care providers and specialists was predicted to be fifty-fifty in managed care organizations, a dramatic change from the one-third primary care versus two-thirds specialists in fee-for-service medicine (Gamliel, Politzer, Rivo, and Mullan, 1995: 134–135).

This surplus also helps to explain why physicians began signing up with multiple managed care plans and discounting their fees. Competition for patients became acute. Although the number of patient visits per person continued to climb into the late 1980s, the number of visits per doctor continued to decline. Access to the flow of patients became critical to doctors in the 1980s and early 1990s, since the government payers, Medicaid and Medicare, often refrained from raising their rates. With cost containment the driving force in the reorganization of the health care system, the selling power of the medical profession was consequently reduced.

The profession was faced with an interesting but painful dilemma: how to maintain its role as the friend, significant service provider, even confidant for patients, when many members of the medical profession were compelled by fear of losing patients to join managed care plans. To join a managed care plan might mean implementing cost-cutting measures, some of which might endanger the lives and well-being of their patients. Protecting the bottom line by limiting medical expenditures became the unwelcome guest during every encounter between doctor and patient. It certainly was a change from previous epochs in the history of the medical profession in America.

REFERENCES

Blumenthal, D. 2001. "Controlling health care expenditures." *New England Journal of Medicine 344* (10)(March 8): 766–69.

Cacioppo, J.C., Diettrich, N.A., Kaplan, G., and Nora, P.F. 1989. "The consequences of current constraints on surgical treatment of appendicitis." *American Journal of Surgery 157* (3)(March): 276–81.

Ellis, F.J. 2000. "Faculty and students turn to business training to fine tune medical practice." *Academic Physician and Scientist* (November/December): 1, 4.

Feldstein, P.J. 1986. "The emergence of market competition in the U.S. health care system: Its causes, likely structure and implications." *Health Policy 6*: 1–20.

Freudenheim, M. 1991. "Health care a growing burden." *New York Times* (January 29): D1, D9.

Gamliel, S., Politzer, R.M., Rivo, M.L., and Mullan, F. 1995. "Managed care on the march: Will physicians meet the challenge?" *Health Affairs 14* (2) (Summer): 131–42.

Howell, J.D. 1999. "The paradox of osteopathy." *New England Journal of Medicine 341* (November 4): 1465–67.

Kahn, K. L., Rubenstein, L.V., Draper, D., Kosecoff, J. Rogers, W.H., Keeler, E.B. and R.H. Brook. 1990. "The effects of the DRG-based prospective payment system on quality of care for hospitalized Medicare patients: An introduction to the series." *Journal of the American Medical Association 264* (15) (October 17): 1953–55.

Krause, E. 1996. *The Death of the Guilds*. New Haven, CT: Yale University Press.

Levit, K.R., Freeland, M.S., and Waldo, D.R. 1989. "Health spending and ability to pay: business, individuals, and government." *Health Care Financing Review 3* (10) (Spring): 1–11.

Pear, R. 2001. "Medicare shift: Doctors' errors to be disclosed." *New York Times* (January 2): A1, A12.

———. 2000. "Ex-enemies on insurance offer a plan that would include half without coverage." Available online at http://www.nytimes.com/2000/11/21/national/21 INSU.html (11/21/2000).

Relman, A. 1991. "Shattuck lecture—The health care industry: Where is it taking us?" *New England Journal of Medicine 325* (12)(September 19): 854–59.

Remler, D.K., Donelan, K., Blendon, R.J., Lundberg, G.D., Leape, L.L., Calkins, D.R., Binns, K., and Newhouse, J.P. 1997. "What do managed care plans do to affect care? Results from a survey of physicians." *Inquiry 34*: 204.

Ritzer, G., and Walczak, D. 1986. "Rationalization and the deprofessionalization of physicians." *Social Forces 67* (1)(September): 1–22.

Roback, G., Randolph, L., and Seidman, B. 1993. *Physician Characteristics and Distribution in the US*. Chicago, IL: American Medical Association.

Rogers, W.H., Draper, D., Kahn, K., Keeler, E.B., Rubenstein, L.V., Kosecoff, J., and Brooks, R.H. 1990. "Quality of care before and after implementation of the DRG-based prospective payment system: A summary of effects." *Journal of the American Medical Association 264* (15)(October 17): 1989–94.

Schroeder, S.A., and Cantor, J.C. 1991. "On squeezing balloons: Cost control fails again." *New England Journal of Medicine 325* (15)(October 10): 1099–100.

Siu, A.L., Manning, W.G., and Benjamin, B. 1990. "Patient, provider, and hospital characteristics associated with inappropriate hospitalization." *American Journal of Public Health 80* (10)(October): 1253-56.

Thurow, L.C. 1984. "Sounding board: Learning to say no." *New England Journal of Medicine 311* (24) (December 13): 1569–71.

Vladeck, B.C. 1990. "Hospitals and the public purse." *Transactions and Studies 7* (2)(June): 263–94.

Weitzman, B.C. 1990. "The quality of care: Assessments and assurances." In Anthony R. Kovner (ed.), *Health Care Delivery in the United States*, 4th ed., 353–80. New York: Springer.

Wickizer, T.M. 1990. "The effect of utilization review on hospital use and expenditures: A review of the literature and an update on recent findings." *Medical Care Review 47* (3)(Fall): 327–63.

2

What's Behind the Changing Doctor-Patient Relationship

The relationship with one's doctor has often been very special for most Americans. Even when Americans say they are losing respect for the medical profession, they often show a great deal of admiration for their doctor(s). Much regret is expressed about how the vast changes that have occurred in the health care system over the past two decades have made that relationship more impersonal and commercial. The feeling of disconsolation is mutual. Arnold Relman (1991), former editor of the *New England Journal of Medicine*, although hardly one to ignore organized medicine's flaws, suggests that the entrance of the profit motive in health care has created a turning point in the relationship between doctor and patient.

The key question is, Will medicine become essentially a business or will it remain a profession? ... Will we act as businessmen in a system that is becoming increasingly entrepreneurial or will we choose to remain a profession with all the obligations for self-regulation and protection of the public interest that this commitment implies?

It is hard to imagine a social relationship, except perhaps those between races and sexes, that has changed more in the past quarter century than the one between doctor and patient. Clinical settings have become filled with various kinds of assistants, available to free the doctor from the routine and the ordinary. And these support personnel represent only the employees who come into direct contact with patients. The

Dictionary of Occupational Titles lists more than 200 health-care jobs. With all this help, a patient might assume the doctor is ready to do what leading studies of communication between doctor and patient consider the essence of the relationship—establish a clinical focus for the medical encounter. Active exchange of information, for example, is necessary to establish the reason for provider-patient contact, the nature of the perceived problem, plans for action, the feasibility of such plans, and the responsibility and acceptance of all parties involved (Inui and Carter, 1985: 522).

Yet patients complain that too often the doctor isn't tuned in. How we interact with doctors reflects some of the major transformations undergone and ongoing in the health-care delivery system, brought about by an evolving financing system, new technology, changing demographics, and efforts to contain costs by restraining utilization.

Almost thirty years ago, a report on the American health-care system was subtitled "Doing Better, Feeling Worse." As we begin a new century, that title is even more appropriate than in the 1970s. The declining percentage of insured Americans in the 1990s notwithstanding, there has never been a time when doctors could do more technically for patients, there have never been so many people who regularly use health-care services, and there have never been so many doctors available to deliver services. Why should so many Americans believe that the current health-care system needs complete reconstruction? How did we come to this situation of widespread dissatisfaction amidst medical progress?

When Richard Nixon was president—the time when the report on the health-care system of the 1970s was being constructed—he expressed an attitude toward government financing of health care that represented the views of many American physicians and a good many ordinary citizens. As a patient, he said, he would rather have the doctor work for him than for the government. Expressing the view that the doctor-patient relationship is sacred and should not be violated in any way, he also avoided taking necessary steps to generate a national health insurance system. Nixon failed to note that there were already a great number of different payers—including Medicare and Medicaid, two government-financed programs—constituting a third party to the doctor-patient relationship.

The Nixon presidency was historically a perfect time to take action. After the Indochina War, better known as the Vietnam War, there was a window of opportunity to create the kind of financing that would create health security for millions of Americans and create a single-payer system that could bargain with providers about charges. An impressive agenda of social legislation was made into law during this period, but universal access to health care did not become part of the Nixon legacy. Unfortunately, ideology prevented such action. Traditional ideas, about medicine as well as other American institutions, are often invoked to protect the controlling interests in these realms.

Hence, although our politicians often imagine and romanticize the past and preserve ideas of unrestricted markets at the expense of economic growth, there is a profound sense in the United States today that relationships with doctors are not satisfactory. Doctors themselves long for the simple days before all the new rules and regulations that impinge on their practice and their relationship with patients.

THE GOLDEN AGE OF AMERICAN MEDICINE

A revisit to the golden age of medicine also sheds light on some of the organizational and cultural supports that were put in place by the profession to gain its sovereignty in American society. The medical expert became recognized as an important provider of support services in a society where, because of interdependence, labor's availability was becoming increasingly important.

In essence, the division of labor, specialization, and the commercial way of life was seen as a seamless system. In many respects, in the age of industrial capitalist development, public health measures were seen as primary and medical diagnosis and treatment as secondary. Medical technology and interventions as weapons used by doctors to directly save lives were limited; they were later deemed by medical historians as mostly ineffective until the development of antibiotics.

The medical profession, despite its limited effectiveness, attempted to provide direct help. It also sought legitimacy, or a kind of popular *and* official recognition of its stature in society. Sociologists and other students of the professions recognize that these claims may be subject to inquiries based on the scholarly or scientific value of organized skepticism. Paul Starr, a contemporary student of the medical profession, provides a clear illustration of this orientation and what must be attended to when examining a profession from a sociological perspective.

Professional claims, of course should not be taken simply on face value. The rewards of professional status encourage would-be and even established professions to invent or elaborate credentials, sciences, and codes of ethics in bids for recognition. Rather than as indicators of professional status, such features should be seen as the means of legitimating solidarity among practitioners and gaining a grant of monopoly from the state. Occupations may or may not succeed, depending on their means of collective organization and the receptivity of the public and the government. In this sense, professionalism represents a form of occupational control rather than a quality that inheres in some kind of work. But professionalism is also a kind of solidarity, a source of meaning in work, and a system of regulating belief in modern society. (Starr, 1982: 16)

Specifically, how did medicine become regarded as a sovereign profession in the United States? There were many milestones. At the beginning of the last century, the medical profession started to take control over the technology and distribution of pharmaceutical products. In the area of knowledge about medications and their use, the profession established its position as the agent of control even before state licensing of physicians became widespread. By setting up the Council on Pharmacy and Chemistry in 1905, the American Medical Association (AMA) sought to lead the struggle against the sale of over-the-counter medications. In so doing, some physicians asserted quite simply that their advice was more important than the written material issued by the manufacturers of nostrums. The reformist spirit against patent medicines was made into association policy. No longer taking advertising in its journal for over-the-counter medications, the AMA, through its council, refused to approve any medication directly advertised to the public as useful in fighting a disease. The AMA physicians sought to become the sole experts on diseases and which medications were to be used to fight them. In establishing these rules and regulations, the AMA successfully won the right to become the institutional linkage between the patient and the drug manufacturer (Starr, 1982: 131–33).

Once medicine's authority was established in these areas, the manufacturers of pharmaceuticals provided advertising revenues for AMA journals, which then were used by the AMA leadership to create uniformity in outlook and social integration in medicine throughout the United States. Funds were strategically allocated to fight dissenters within the profession. As Starr notes in his social history of American medicine, the AMA knew how to use its power to attain these goals.

In 1912 the AMA set up a cooperative advertising bureau, which channeled advertisements to state medical journals. The bureau gave the AMA considerable financial leverage over the state medical societies and helped bind the national association even more tightly together. Once again cultural authority was being converted into economic power and effective political organization (Starr, 1982: 134).

Later, after World War II, in response to the Truman administration's efforts to establish a national health insurance program, these same sources of funds were used to help the AMA keep its power.

Organized medicine received large contributions from pharmaceutical firms to fight health insurance, in addition to the revenues from pharmaceutical advertising in AMA journals. The doctors received this support in part because of the strategic location they held in the marketing of drugs; their gatekeeping functions allowed them to collect a toll for use in political agitation. (Starr, 1982: 288)

Following licensing and the reform of medical education, there may have been a "new morning" in American medicine, but since then, other eras characterized by uncontrolled spending have ensued. Now new concerns, voiced by our industrial and commercial chieftains, with declining productivity and profits, have come to the foreground, suggesting that employee and dependent health care take up too great a part of all their expenses. In addition, some observers, and part of the general public as well, think the profession of medicine is guided by an all-consuming interest in income, protection from malpractice suits, and thoughtless use of technology instead of good judgment. The patient loses out in this setting, becoming depersonalized while being helped.

Although doctors have been around for millennia, they have not always been regarded as essential for society. Over the ages, dramatists have often expressed their disdain for the medical arts, and doctors have been subject to ridicule in fiction because of their ineptitude as well as feared for their technical skills. That rich compendium of our evolving language, the *Dictionary of American Slang*, includes expressions such as "quack," "sawbones," and "croaker," and reminds us how medical practitioners were denigrated in the nineteenth century. The increased status and power of the profession paralleled the historical changes of industrialization and the increasing division of labor in society.

By the first quarter of the twentieth century, however, medical doctors were not only praised as the guardians of the common good, but also esteemed as savers of lives through their direct intervention. During that progressive era, the American Medical Association even advocated national health insurance, a position it has since abandoned during its conservative years. Even thirty-five years ago, admiration for doctors was so strong that in a social science journal article, Myerhoff and Larson (1965: 188) depicted them as compassionate experts—indeed culture heroes—not just because they dealt with life and death but because they were interpreters in the face of uncertainty, defining "the ingredients of typical situations, depicting appropriate behavior and accompanying motivations and interpretations."

For those who could afford them as a regular source of care, doctors were attentive, courteous, and warm. In an age when physicians depended on a limited market for their services, they had to demonstrate their devotion to the few patients they had. They wished to retain patients as much as possible, and they wanted their patients to say good things about them in their neighborhoods, churches, and clubs. By keeping their fees low, doctors sought to cast as wide a net as possible to capture paying patients. In fact, general practitioners were reluctant to part with a patient through a referral to a specialist if they thought they could continue to help. Naturally, specialists knew this and expressed a great deal of gratitude for a referral because it was so hard-won.

These arrangements worked to establish medicine as the major provider of health-care services to the middle classes in the United States and promote the development of the modern acute-care voluntary hospital, as we know it today (Rosenberg, 1987). By the 1930s this system was threatened as the middle classes' purchasing power declined. During the Great Depression, patients could pay neither their hospital nor their doctor bills. To keep voluntary hospital beds filled and their doors open, group hospital insurance policies were underwritten and premiums collected from subscribers. Usually, these policies were available to a workforce, such as schoolteachers, that expected to be steadily employed. Blue Cross hospital insurance was developed by the hospital industry itself as a way to keep generating income during those gloomy days.

What worked in a mutually advantageous way for provider and consumer alike during hard times proved even more popular during good times, when more people wished to share in the good life. But when first introduced, group policies were used as a way of keeping valued workers happy. Health insurance policies were offered as an across-the-board fringe benefit during World War II, when wage and price freezes, compounded by a labor shortage, made it hard to retain employees without offering some reward. Then, during the postwar 1940s and 1950s, an era of substantial increases in real earnings and high progressive taxation, unionized workers sought to gain health benefits in collective bargaining agreements, sometimes in preference to increases in wages because they were considered untaxed income.

The health insurance industry was off and running now, and health-care providers were beneficiaries. Hospital bills were paid by insurance policies, and it was not too long before major medical care was also covered by indemnification policies. Benefits permitted potential patients and their providers to interact more; some of the real financial barriers to receiving medical care had come down.

Insurance had major consequences in changing the behavior of patients and their doctors. Consistently, studies have shown that insured patients are greater users of care when it is possible to control for type of illness. Known as third-party payers, private insurance coverage made it possible for patients to seek doctors with great frequency, resulting in larger patient panels, or rosters, and more appointments per day. In fact, under these new financial conditions, which produced more patient volume, general practitioners were less reluctant to refer to specialists.

The presence of coverage enhanced doctor-patient contact. For patients, insurance protected their assets because their bills were paid; for doctors, whose operating costs were more or less fixed, it meant more income as each additional patient seen during the day resulted in an increasingly profitable consultation. Moreover, access to specialists was no longer restricted by economic considerations. Each referral was less essential to specialists' practices, but, as with general practitioners, more economically valuable than in the past.

Although third-party payment augments, but does not replace, the classic fee-for-service relationship between doctors and patients, it still means some out-of-pocket costs for routine office visits. The concept of insurance was a way to protect against major economic catastrophes that could befall a family, such as the death of the major wage earner, or the loss of a home or business. Some consumers and a few providers became concerned about the high cost of services rendered. Models for how to rein in out-of-pocket expenditures did exist, although the American Medical Association severely disapproved of doctors who worked for a salary—the keystone of these groups that provided comprehensive care for a single fee paid up front. Kaiser and other early health maintenance organizations delivered good services at moderate cost to the membership. Through this prepayment arrangement with specific providers, consumers "locked in" their health care costs for an entire year. Not only were doctors' services available under these plans, but hospital care was also included for a single fee, with the provider assuming the financial risk if there was disproportionately high patient utilization of their services.

Ever since the 1930s, patients and employers concerned about controlling their expenditures for health care have sought ways of fixing their payments before they use the services. Leadership in this area came from progressive industrialist Henry J. Kaiser, who protected employees and their families from excessive health-care expenses, first in the construction of the Grand Coulee Dam, and later in the World War II–driven shipbuilding industry. At the work site of this great public works project of the depression era, a small amount was deducted from the pay of the construction workers to cover care provided by a doctor and his portable infirmary. From these humble origins, health maintenance organizations (HMOs) evolved.

Today in HMO programs, a group of doctors, including specialists, provide all the medical specialties and services by contract to a number of patients who will be cared for, no matter how frequently or infrequently they use the services. Hospital-based services are also part of the benefits and are prearranged by contracts between HMOs and hospitals or by outright purchase or building of hospitals dedicated exclusively to caring for subscribers. Described as "prepaid" or "capitation" payment plans, HMOs are a way of financing care as well as organizing and delivering services. Few patients who contracted for these services complained that they had little control over doctors because they did not pay them directly, a claim often made by true believers in fee-for-service medicine. If anything, since they paid no additional fees for them and believed that they had rights to specialty care by contract, patients were more demanding of services, particularly diagnostic tests (Freidson, 1975).

Recognizing this problem, some contemporary HMOs provide financial incentives to primary-care physicians to keep expenses down by constraining diagnostic testing and the use of specialty care (Abramson, 1990). Surely all these changes in the financing and delivery of medical services have altered the relationship between patients and physicians. With little incentive to spend time with the patient, and with patient panels being far larger than their 1920s counterparts, physicians are less willing or able to get to know patients in depth. In addition, up to the 1960s, a substantial part of general practice consisted of the house call, an occasion where physicians got to know something about the way patients lived (Rothman, 1991). With the advent of insurance and HMO membership plans, Americans were more likely to have a regular source of care, but one that was less familiar with their lifestyles, aspirations, and anxieties. In addition, the tight scheduling of office visits does not permit casual conversation wherein patients might divulge something that is of great concern, permitting them to gain relief or seek advice.

NEW TECHNOLOGY AND OLD RELATIONSHIPS

Increasingly, medicine has relied on sophisticated technology to enhance diagnosis or aid in treatment. Along with this development of new technology is the fact that the gap between what the doctor knows and communicates and what the patient knows and receives grows greater, despite easy access to information (and misinformation) on the Internet. Moreover, medical services are usually offered by one physician to many patients, and care often involves a team of professionals, making the use of time and place a crucial factor in getting things done. Organizational objectives, commonly expressed in the form of productivity or maximized use of facilities, can become more important than a particular patient's need to receive an explanation for why a procedure is being performed. When one becomes a patient, according to the sardonic Erving Goffman (1961), one is made into a "serviceable object." As a result, this great sociologist suggested, a patient—not a person—fits into the existing organizational scheme of things. The results of this process can vary: Sometimes patients feel they are not esteemed, and on rare occasion real harm can occur, as when patients receive the wrong procedure as a result of their providers' devotion to organizational objectives. From the perspective of patients or their guardians, contact with physicians has the potential for leaving them feeling that they are not being treated as people. Contact with medical professionals can reduce the patients' sense of control over their own lives. This outcome is a reversal of the motivation for going to the doctor, an occasion that is meant to increase a person's power over his or her life. It can be resented bitterly.

Leon Eisenberg, a psychiatrist, expresses the importance of this moment of empowerment:

The doctor's task ought still to be to educate the patient about the meaning of the illness and the methods for its remedy, after he has learned the patient's conception of its cause and how it might be treated. The process is one of exchange of information, the goal is the demystification of medical procedures, so that the patient is able to make his own decisions and thereby assume responsibility for acting. (1977: 237)

Although great progress has been made in health-care technology, social skills are necessary to get patients to discuss their symptoms and follow treatment regimens. Communication involves responding to patients as well as directing them. On many occasions, informed patients do not understand the nature of the diagnosis or their prognosis. According to Goleman (1991), sociolinguist Richard Frankel analyzed a thousand letters from dissatisfied patients at a large Michigan health maintenance organization. He concluded that 90 percent of the complaints related to the communication styles of medical staff. Among these complaints was the use of medical terminology that confused patients. Moreover, failure to look at patients during the encounter was seen as part of the physician's lack of compassion for the patient. Words and gestures both need to be considered when giving serious news to patients.

Frankel has also analyzed directly the interaction between patients and physicians. He found that in more than half of the seventy-four medical interviews he studied, patients were interrupted by the physicians within eighteen seconds of beginning to explain what had brought them to the doctor's office. Failure to allow patients to express their thoughts can lead to termination of the relationship and even poor compliance with the treatment regimen. For most chronic illnesses the model for doctor-patient relationships has been conceptualized as involving guidance from the provider and patient cooperation (Szasz and Hollander, 1956). More recent studies on the health outcomes of diabetics, people with hypertension, and those with ulcers demonstrated that patients' conditions improved when they were allowed to bring up everything they wished in discussions with their doctors (Goleman, 1991). When internists monitored patients, those patients who gained more control over their situation performed better in later checkups. Diabetics who participated strongly in their examination showed a clinically significant 15 percent decrease in blood sugar levels two months later.

Given the destination, or direction in which the technological imperative is taking medicine, these observations on the need for communication are not surprising. New diagnostic and treatment techniques look for hard signs of disease and limit the need to identify the more subjective responses or symptoms that clinicians relied on to diagnose disease or determine whether progress or deterioration was occurring in a patient's condition. Communication seems to be the key to good relationships between providers and patients and good care, but current trends diminish the possibility of mutually satisfying interchanges. Doctors frequently interrupt patients to move the diagnostic process along. Yet patients need to tell their story. Meanwhile, the diagnostic equipment remains idle.

Some interesting questions remain. Will patients be allowed to discuss their illnesses during a consultation when it does not inform the physician in any medically necessary way? How can patients gain control over a situation in which the diagnosis is performed by a machine?

Outside of immunizations, new technology means greater profits for their manufacturers so long as their products are accepted as a standard tool in the doctor's arsenal. Manufacturers of diagnostic equipment, monitoring devices, and pharmaceuticals all need to get the real consumer (i.e., the physician) to use their products. Getting these products accepted involves efforts of persuasion comparable to selling to any target audience of consumers. The manufacturers have a built-in advantage, given the nature of medical practice in the United States. Physicians were, up to the advent of managed care, more highly rewarded, both materially and professionally, for performing procedures than for engaging in educational efforts with patients. Third-party payers regard these procedures as more complex than patient education and reimburse claims more handsomely when technology is used. In addition, the more procedures performed with physician-owned diagnostic equipment, the more financially rewarding these procedures are. Recent studies point to differences in the use of diagnostic equipment according to ownership by the examining physician. Moreover, the task can usually be delegated to a technician who can gain proficiency at doing it unsupervised while the physician is doing other things. Reporting in 1991, the Florida Health Care Cost Containment Board, a state agency, found that when doctors owned their own laboratories, almost twice as many tests were performed for each patient as at other laboratories. In this comprehensive study of the Sunshine State, similar results were found for frequency of scheduled visits to physical therapy centers that were owned in joint ventures by doctors (*New York Times*, August 11, 1991: E9). According to the report, 45 percent of the state's doctors were involved in such arrangements and more than 90 percent of the diagnostic imaging centers in Florida were wholly or partly owned by doctors

The Florida report also concluded that poor and rural residents did not have improved access to these diagnostic and clinical services. This kind of finding is not limited to areas where senior citizens abound. Another recent statewide study of almost 38,000 patients at 100 hospitals, reported in the *Journal of the American Medical Association*, found that patients with the same symptoms receive more diagnostic testing when they are covered by insurance than when they are not (Wenneker, 1990). Massachusetts patients with chest pains or circulatory problems who were insured were more likely to receive a diagnosis for, or be treated for, heart disease than patients without insurance or those who were covered by Medicaid. Equipment and staff time is sometimes used selectively so that the procedures ordered will yield revenues. Similarly, patients who are Medicaid-eligible yield lower returns for the same diagnostic procedures than those who are insured or covered by the Medicare program, and also receive less testing.

Paralleling the extension of technology as part of the relationship with patients was the development of life-extending technology for those near death. Respirators were originally designed for and used with patients who had lung surgery, allowing these organs to recover slowly. Additional uses were found in intensive care units for this equipment, and patients with multiple organ failures who were in critical condition were placed on respirators.

Following the scholarly exposé in a major medical journal on involuntary clinical experimentation initiated by Beecher (1966), in which he cited numerous studies in which patients never gave informed consent to participate in dangerous experiments, federal legislators and patients' rights advocates began to wonder how much choice patients had in undergoing clinical procedures or treatment regimens that might be futile, invasive, or have adverse side effects. The development of informed consent for standard clinical care followed on the heels of similar protocols to protect the rights of subjects in experiments. It is not surprising that consumers began to wonder whether they were being told everything, or whether doctors knew how to communicate with patients.

CHANGING DEMOGRAPHICS

All these changes in financing, technology, and concern for patients' rights were intensified by the enormous increase in access to medical care for the elderly through Medicare and the general aging of the population. With fewer children being born, the proportion of elderly increased, making for an older population. And clearly, older people have more health problems per individual than younger ones.

The bicentennial year 1976 witnessed not only a celebration of the birth of the United States, but the end of a time when more than half the population was under the age of 30. Although the median age in 1977

was 28.9, it is anticipated that by the year 2030 more than half the population will be over 36 (Reinhold, 1977: 1). As a consequence of this
change in demographics, physicians are treating more patients with
chronic diseases (especially heart disease and cancer) and fewer with
acute diseases (such as pneumonia). Increasingly, these kinds of cases
require many outpatient visits and less need for hospitalization.

To make up for the increasing demand for services, medical schools
made a great effort in the 1970s to expand the supply of doctors in the
United States. Physician extenders such as physician's assistants and
nurse practitioners were also created to make up for the lack of primary-
care doctors. Additionally, foreign medical school graduates came to the
United States in large numbers. Although their pass rate on the national
foreign medical school examination was low, the sheer volume of doctors
trained outside the country who took the examination helped swell the
ranks of licensed practitioners in the United States. The presence of so
many doctors has increased access but also increased health-care expenditures in the past decade.

Health-policy experts have often observed that in the current decade
there is an oversupply of physicians, particularly specialists. Compared
with other countries with similar standards of living and life expectancy,
we depend far more on specialty care than on general or family practice
medicine. Increasingly, Americans with insurance coverage, including
Medicaid or Medicare, have easy access to medical care. (The quality of
the care is rarely considered an issue.) This situation is not without adverse consequences, mainly the increasing expenditures on health care.
Accessible services for some promotes unnecessary utilization as much
as it does adequate availability of care. Modern medicine has an activist
orientation, a cultural value that promotes intervention even when marginally useful or not especially in the patient's best interest. Unnecessary
surgery, for example, can lead to avoidable deaths from infection, excessive anesthesia, or other complications. For patients on a dying trajectory,
the use of expensive and invasive technology may produce extremely
limited positive results. Finally, it has often been noted that most of one's
lifetime medical expenditures are incurred during the last three months
of life. Even during the age of managed care, the 1996 Medical Expen-
diture Panel Survey (MEPS) reported a skewed concentration of expenditures. Only 5 percent of the population accounts for the majority of
health expenditures (Berk and Monheit, 2001). Modern data acquisition
and analysis suggests the policy question for decision makers in the
United States: What are we going to do about this disproportionate distribution of expensive technology and labor? Once reviewed, information
of this kind cannot remain buried in technical reports, published or un-
published.

THE GROWTH OF INFORMATION TECHNOLOGY (IT)

The information technology revolution wants us whether we want it or not. Many people would like it to go away. There is a standing joke in my family concerning the Birenbaums' limited access to modern technology. The room where the computer sits, with its Internet connection by ancient telephone modem, is designated the "IT room." But information technology is no joke. The health-care industry is heavily invested in it. Health care is now watched more closely by cost-conscious corporations and insurers than episodes of *The Sopranos* or *Seinfeld* reruns are viewed by the American public.

The use or misuse of resources in the health-care industry influences decisions on the managerial level of the organization. Documentation of these occurrences in hospitals was once conducted one case at a time by mortality review procedures. Computers make data collection and analysis far easier than in the past. Monitoring of care now is done in more cases and not just to protect the patient's life and health. In fact, the computer-age technology that makes it possible to do many of the diagnostic procedures on patients also permits studies of outcomes, excessive utilization, and different practice styles among the same kind of specialists.

Given that caregivers are studied even more closely than patients, the potential for feeding back information to get doctors to change their practices is certainly present. However, reeducation has demonstrated inconsistent results. Health-policy experts and payers consider that the overuse of services produces excessive costs to payers and patients alike and has introduced various programs to restrain unnecessary utilization.

This strategy focuses on avoiding certain outcomes rather than dealing globally with reforming medical education, reorganizing medical-care resources, or restructuring the payment system. Few schemes to save money attempt to limit the supply of specialty care providers—the great consumers of technology—or expand access to primary care. Rather, the experts who advocate managed care seek to control patient behavior (networks of providers), medical-care organizations (HMOs), or practice styles (authorization). With annual costs for insurance per employee and family dependents now averaging more than $6,348 a year, huge savings can be realized if resource-utilization patterns can be altered (Schroeder, 2001). As of 1999, 91 percent of all members of employer-sponsored health plans had some form of managed care arrangement, an increase of 18 percent from 1996 (Heffler et al., 2001: 197).

The most essential form of managed care involves networks of providers (that is, hospitals and doctors) who discount fees for employees of firms that develop these arrangements. Employees pay a lower co-payment or none at all when they use a member of the network or what is also known as a preferred-provider organization (PPO). Health maintenance organizations are also considered to be forms of managed care because they provide ways of establishing comprehensive services, which restrict access to diagnostic testing, use of specialty care, and hospitalization. Health maintenance organizations attempt to keep people well by focusing a great deal on the prevention of illness (immunization) and early detection, such as Pap smears.

Needless to say, relationships with physicians have become very complex. Patients with real problems are in a quandary as to whether to use or avoid a network. Some physicians belong to many networks at the same time to cast as wide a net as possible. This arrangement may work for patients who are basically healthy and not suffering from a serious chronic illness. One of the problems with these networks is that not every doctor belongs to them. Therefore, patients with serious chronic illnesses who wish to join the network may have to give up a relationship with a doctor who is thoroughly familiar with their medical history. Losing a good cardiologist who has managed *directly* the care of someone after a heart attack but is not part of the network may be an aggravating decision for a person with heart disease, but many patients now give up those specialists with whom they have a good relationship to control or reduce their out-of-pocket expenditures. When people switch plans, albeit reluctantly, they are attempting to control their lives and adapt to changing circumstances. The alternative is to put up with unaffordable medical expenses, a situation that can also contribute to a person's anxiety, elevating blood pressure and producing other unwanted results.

Doctors also are worried about these new programs that seek to contain costs. The managed-care concept has been extended to the review of clinical decision making. Considered a form of second-guessing by some irate providers, it is designed to reduce unnecessary services, or the use of ineffective procedures. It certainly makes relations with patients contingent on the plan to which they belong. One plan may approve a procedure for a patient within a particular disease category, whereas another may not approve the same procedure for a different patient in the same disease category.

None of this kind of managed care would be possible without health-services research data, which is collected widely throughout the United States. Using data on differential rates of treatment, surgery, and diagnosis by practitioners, hospital-related infections, complications, and deaths, employers and insurers decide what to pay for or where to seek services.

Often managed-care information is collected and used by review companies that require preapproval for procedures covered by insurers.

Nurses employed by a review company—Value Health Sciences, for example—match symptoms with proposed treatment regimens. When a match occurs, approval is granted to the provider and the patient, and the procedure is paid for by the insurance company. If there is no match, referral is made to a physician adviser employed by this review company. A negotiation process between the clinician and the adviser usually follows on the heels of the denial of authorization, a time-consuming and sometimes irritating process.

Physicians complain that their professional autonomy is destroyed by these review procedures. But review organizations also depend upon physicians to construct protocols and advise providers about alternatives if requests are denied. Why was this not possible thirty-five years ago? During the gravy years, doctors were more likely to stick together and close ranks when faced by government action or insurance company rulings. The current physician surplus makes it possible for review companies to fill these jobs. Although some unnecessary procedures may be avoided, the presence of as many as 300 managed-care organizations, each with different rules and regulations, means that practicing doctors navigate in a very different environment. It also means that they must become very sophisticated about who is covered by what.

This lack of uniformity in care introduced by monitoring and permission systems affects relationships between doctors and their patients. Not only is there a third-party payer, but that partner in the relationship hires experts who are able to question the doctor's judgment concerning the effectiveness and safety of procedures. It comes as no surprise that these relationships with reviewing companies are sometimes called the "fourth party."

Utilization review organizations present new hurdles for doctors. They sometimes attempt to get around the review procedures by deception. Called "gaming" by both provider and payer, network participants may seek to upgrade diagnoses or the presence of symptoms to gain permission to do a diagnostic procedure. To get around the rules they may suggest that the patient has a co-morbidity, a second sickness, that limits certain kinds of treatment and calls for others. Providers may also schedule extra visits to make up for losses taken through discounting or accepting the assigned rate by the payer.

There are some humorous sides to this contest. Gaming can be tricky for doctors when they do not keep up with the patient's latest change of employment. Patients now change insurance coverage frequently, and doctors may seek to gain remuneration from a plan that no longer covers the patient. When insurance fails to pay a claim, the doctor is not the only one who learns about these efforts at gaming. Patients may discover that the doctor is billing for a visit that never took place or for treating a disease they never had.

Ironically, managed care is somewhat of an unanticipated consequence of federal regulatory efforts to control health care expenditures in the United States. Rules introduced by public regulatory authorities, such as the Health Systems Agency or the Health Care Financing Administration, or by private insurance companies to reduce hospital admissions and length of stay, have increased the number of procedures performed on an outpatient basis and consequently have forced insurers and employers to look for ways to contain these costs. When doctors started doing surgery in outpatient facilities, they increased their fees to compensate for the loss of income resulting from doing fewer inpatient procedures.

Managed care means, in sum, that there are more people looking over the doctor's shoulder. These practices are controversial in two ways: (1) Although they may save some dollars on fees for service, review organizations run up overhead expenses for the insurance companies (fees of review companies) and providers as well (the cost in time and money in generating documentation), and (2) there are some serious concerns on the part of doctors that managed care may negatively affect patient care.

In a humorous article with serious import, Gerald Grumet (1989), a Rochester, New York, physician, claims that managed care rations health care through inconvenience. Consequently, health care is simply doled out more slowly than in the past. He suggests that inconvenience is the third party's secret weapon, involving procedural complexities for filing claims that shift all the time, with each payer using a unique set of exotic terms, slowing down the outflow of funds with various fail-safe mechanisms. This rule-ridden payment maze is unique to a multiple-payer health-care system, compounded by the existence of overlapping coverage, and further fractured by the unbundling of claims to different departments at the same paying agency or private insurance carrier. The result is a great deal of uncertainty for the provider as well as the patient as to what is covered and when they will be paid or reimbursed. Certainly this is not a way to boost morale when treating the sick. Perhaps the new culture heroes of our time are the health-policy analysts and researchers, who can try to explain it all and give us certainty in the face of uncertainty. I am waiting to see the first HBO pilot, starring Glenn Close as a savvy School of Public Health professor called in to calm distressed subscribers to insurance plans or HMOs when they feel they are being denied help. (Before I could pitch this idea to the premium channels, Laura Dern played the whistle-blowing doctor in the film "Mangled Care" on the Showtime channel, made available to viewers in May 2002.)

MANAGED CARE, PATIENT TRUST, AND PSYCHIATRIC SERVICES

A good case study of how managed care can cause distress exists in the field of mental health. To be sure, underutilization of mental health services preceded the conversion of health insurance to managed care. By virtue of the fact that insurers did not cover mental illness in the same way that they covered physical illness, people suffering from mental disease did not seek out services. Other barriers to access relate to the stigma associated with mental illness. A person with such an illness is sometimes devalued in the eyes of others.

Psychiatry and other mental health services are particularly vulnerable to managed-care concepts. First, many of the symptoms of psychiatric illness may be seen in the popular view as moral weakness and therefore not in need of treatment. Second, anyone who gets to play the sick role is often suspected of malingering to get them to give up the comfort and rewards of being treated as a person with unwanted problems, and the person with psychiatric symptoms may be seen as doing just that. Third, even advocates of clinical care recognize that outcome studies where psychiatric hospitalization is involved are needed.

In dealing with mental illness (for example, depression) and behavioral health issues such as drug addiction, the field of psychiatry and its patients have been strongly subjected to managed care plan review, as will be shown in greater detail in Chapter 3. Inarguably, in no area of medicine have managed-care components of insurance policies created more controversy than in psychiatric hospitalization. Not only do psychiatrists regard the intervention of managed-care companies in determining whether or not payment of long-term hospitalization will continue as irrational as well as adversarial, but they have argued in their own journals that such interference is harmful to patients' recovery. There is great concern among mental health providers that patients may be discharged too soon, against their best professional judgment. If doctors take an oath to do no harm, perhaps managed-care companies, built around the use of medical expertise, need to be sworn in as well to avoid *underutilization* as well as overutilization of services.

In all fairness to the insurance companies and their reviewers, the focus of these refusals to authorize certain stays in hospital followed the development of private for-profit psychiatric hospitals, which were suspected of providing custodial rather than therapeutic care. In some states, private psychiatric hospitals offered bounties for patients, violating the rights of ordinary citizens to due process in the course of an involuntary commitment. In some instances, moreover, reviewers and providers were able to work cooperatively for the patient's best interest.

In general, however, insurers suspect that psychiatric treatment, whether for inpatient or outpatient care, is less valuable than care for physical illness. This bias is adopted by some employers who want to save money on health insurance for employees and their families. Bias-based cost cutting may be counterproductive, since there is evidence that counseling services for workers reduce the number of days lost through sickness or absenteeism. Finally, the failure to deal with psychiatric illness does not mean the problem will resolve itself. Untreated psychiatric illness has its costs to society and significant others, and there is always the possibility of the intrapsychic stress manifesting itself in the form of physical illness or suicidal behavior. Unfortunately, psychiatric assessments and treatments are not considered primary or secondary preventions.

THE END OF THE GOLDEN AGE OF MEDICINE

The golden age of medicine lasted quite a long time. There were some snakes in the medical Garden of Eden, although most of them were found on the official symbol of the profession—the staff of Aesculapius. There were some early harbingers of change. Federal support for the development of managed care organizations found in the Health Maintenance Organization Act of 1973 created organizational alternatives to fee-for-service medicine. The American Medical Association was strongly against aid and comfort to HMOs and believed that nonmedical organizations should not be given control over medical services (Bauman, 1976).

Despite all the warnings, the medical profession did quite well financially, even into the late 1980s. Physician income between 1982 and 1989 grew by 24 percent. Although it contributed to concern among health-policy analysts, government officials, and employers, it hardly led to complaints among those reaping the benefits (Pope and Schneider, 1992).

Extensive market penetration by HMOs produced in those metropolitan regions fewer hours worked per year ($-$ 4 percent), 13.7 percent fewer patients seen per week, and higher levels of dissatisfaction ($+$ 20 percent) among the 4,373 patient care physicians under the age of forty-five who were selected through a random sample. Thus, the greater the market penetration by HMOs, the more constraints on practice expressed (Hadley and Mitchell, 1997).

The managed care industry was regarded by physicians in general, not just those in metropolitan areas with high market penetration, as a threat to their autonomy. David C. Colby, an official of the national Physician Payment Review Commission (PPRC), reported in 1997 on a survey conducted by National Opinion Research Center for the commission that

72 percent of physicians said that external review and limitation on clinical decision making were very serious or somewhat serious problems when dealing with HMOs. By contrast, about 50 percent of physicians said that about fee-for-service plans, PPOs, traditional Medicare and Medicaid. (Colby, 1997: 113)

Market conditions also induced some physician practices to merge or affiliate with other practices and hospitals, as uncovered by the Gallup Organization poll conducted for the PPRC. In this 1994 national survey, the researchers found that 19 percent of physicians reported that their practices experienced these major changes (Colby, 1997: 113).

The Gallup survey also asked respondents what the future will be like for physicians. Colby clearly suggests that these results mark the end of the golden age.

Reflecting their loss of dominance and autonomy, physicians believe that others will be extremely important actors in influencing the organization of medicine. Sixty-five percent predicted that insurance companies will be extremely important in shaping the future organization of medicine; 53 percent, large employers; and 52 percent, the government. By contrast, only 30 percent thought physicians would be extremely important (Colby, 1997: 113).

How did this state of affairs come to be? How did it arise that there are these fourth parties looking over the doctor's shoulder? What challenges do they create for providers? How does their presence affect the trust needed to sustain the doctor-patient relationship? In the next chapter I will look at the origins of this development and the consequences for the profession of medicine and begin to tell the tale of the loss of sovereignty for the medical profession.

REFERENCES

Abramson, Leonard. 1990. *Healing Our Health Care System*. New York: Grove Weidenfeld.

Bauman, P. 1976. "The formulation and evolution of the Health Maintenance Organization policy." *Social Science and Medicine* (April-May): 129–42.

Beecher, H.K. 1966. "Consent in clinical experimentation: Myth and reality." *Journal of the American Medical Association 195* (January 3): 34-35.

Berk, M.L., and Monheit, A.C. 2001. "The concentration of health care expenditures revisited." *Health Affairs 20* (2) (March/April): 9–32.

Colby, D.C. 1997. "Perspective: Doctors and their discontents." *Health Affairs 16* (November/December): 112–14.

Eisenberg, Leon. 1977. "The search for care." *Daedalus* (Winter): 235-46.

Freidson, Eliot. 1975. *Doctoring Together: A Study of Professional Control*. New York: Elsevier.

Hadley, J., and Mitchell, J.M. 1997. "Effects of HMO market penetration on physicians' work effort and satisfaction." *Health Affairs* 16 (November/December): 99–111.

Goffman, Erving. 1961. "The medical model and mental hospitalization: Some notes on the vicissitudes of the tinkering trades." In *Asylums: Essays on the Social Situation of Mental Patients and Other Inmates*, pp. 321–86. Garden City, NY: Doubleday Anchor.

Goleman, Daniel. 1991. "All too often the doctor isn't listening, studies show." *New York Times* (November 13): C1, C15.

Grumet, Gerald W. 1989. "Sounding board: Health care rationing through inconvenience." *New England Journal of Medicine* 321 (9) (August 31): 607-11.

Heffler, S., Levit, K., Smith, S., Smith, C., Cowan, C., Lazenby, H., and Freeland, M. 2001. "Trends: Health spending growth up in 1999; faster growth expected in the future." *Health Affairs* 20 (2) (March/April): 193–203.

Inui, T., and Carter, W.B. 1985. "Problems and prospects for health services research on provider-patient communication." *Medical Care* 23 (5) (May): 521-38.

Myerhoff, B., and Larson, W.R. 1965. "The doctor as culture hero: The routinization of charisma." *Human Organization* 24 (3): 188-91.

Pope, G.C., and Schneider, J.E. 1992. "Trends in physician income." *Health Affairs* 11 (Spring): 181–93.

Reinhold, R. 1977. "New population trends transforming U.S." *New York Times* (February 6): 1, 42.

Relman, A. 1991. "Shattuck lecture—The health care industry: where is it taking us?" *New England Journal of Medicine* 331 (7): 471–72.

Rosenberg, Charles. 1987. *The Care of Strangers: The Rise of America's Hospital System.* New York: Basic Books.

Rothman, David J. 1991. *Strangers at the Bedside: A History of How Law and Bioethics Transformed Medical Decision Making.* New York: Basic Books.

Schroeder, S. 2001. "Prospects for expanding health insurance coverage." *New England Journal of Medicine* 344 (1) (March 15): 847–52

Starr, P. 1982. *The Social Transformation of American Medicine: The Rise of a Sovereign Profession and the Making of a Vast Industry.* New York: Basic Books.

Szasz, T.S., and Hollander, M.H. 1956. "A contribution to the philosophy of medicine: The basic models of the doctor-patient relationship." *American Medical Association Archives of Internal Medicine* 97 (May): 585-92.

Wenneker, M.B. 1990. "The association of payer with utilization of cardiac procedures in Massachusetts." *Journal of the American Medical Association* 264 (10) (September 12): 1255-60.

"When doctors own their own labs." *New York Times* (August 11, 1991): E9.

3

Driving Down Costs and Professional Autonomy

The growth of the Internet is the worldwide commercial story of the last years of the twentieth century, but without this remarkable technology the business story of our time could easily be the transformation of the American health care system. This makeover was achieved in a brief period of time and involved a major shift in how health care and the health care system are financed, organized, and practiced. Driven by concerns about cost, beginning in the 1980s corporate purchasers of health care plans demanded that insurers offer alternatives to indemnity payment and fee-for-service arrangements. In response, insurers or self-financed benefits programs created health plans that take advantage of the oversupply of doctors, diagnostic equipment, and hospital beds and received favorable prices for services used. To render even more savings through reduced utilization, health care plans are now micromanaging physician clinical practices.

Be careful what you wish for, Americans: Competition has its limits. Market-driven health care has generated unwanted consequences, including the abandonment of quality care standards, decreased clinical autonomy, and limited access to resources for providers. The popular fear of the early Clinton years, that government-led reform would restrict the freedom of doctors to make medical decisions and patients to choose their providers, is past. Today, change is driven by the marketplace. It is most obvious in the widespread indifference among buyers of care to the plight of the uninsured and the embarrassment of providers who can no longer afford to cross-subsidize uncompensated care for the uninsured. Managers of delivery systems are expected to practice cost containment, not give away services. Investor ownership of managed care plans has created an environment in which providers are more scrutinized than dimpled ballots in Florida.

As far back as the 1920s and 1930s, the economic organization of medicine was subject to review. A national body—the 1927–32 Committee on the Costs of Medical Care—advocated restructuring medicine along lines consistent with its economic environment by integrating the delivery system in a fashion similar to that of an inclusive corporation. The American Medical Association's representatives on the committee dissented, preferring to continue with the status quo, an individual entrepreneurial approach (Perkins, 1998: 1721).

Providers and insured patients today have to be concerned about how markets affect their fortunes. Arnold Relman, the former editor of the esteemed *New England Journal of Medicine*, wrote in 1996 that our brief and abortive period of government-led health-care reform (1993–94) was gentle and kind compared with what has happened.

Ironically, the relatively unregulated, business-dominated market that has taken control of health care since the defeat of the Clinton plan is proving to be a far greater threat to the autonomy of the medical profession than the elaborate apparatus of the plan could ever have been. (p. 601)

The threat to autonomy has also been accompanied by a ratcheting down of fees paid to providers. The groundwork was laid in the 1970s by federal legislation, as shown in Chapter 2. But there was no way to predict back then that market forces would become dominant. Physicians were not prepared for the new world of managed care. Since the 1990s, doctors have been experiencing a loss of power, status, and income. Let the provider beware!

The enormous changes of the last ten years have affected patients, too. Patients may think their physicians are trustworthy but not trust the organizations they work for. David Mechanic and Mark Schlesinger captured the meaning of this concept in their 1996 article on social trust in health-care organizations. They argued that "the success of medical care depends most importantly on patients' trust that their physicians are competent, take appropriate responsibility and control and give their patients' welfare the highest priority" (p. 1693). Now, that trust has been called into question, a result of decisions by employers to reverse the inflationary trends of the 1980s regarding health-care benefits. By 1995–96, inflation in the health care industry had shrunk to close to zero (U.S. Department of Labor, 1996), largely because of a major shift in thinking by benefits officers in large corporations about how much to pay and how to pay for health insurance for employees and their families. These decision makers bet their jobs, or at least their year-end bonuses and stock options, that managed care would produce the dramatic results they wanted.

The early 1990s was "drive time" for benefits managers, and the public was listening to all HMOs options on the radio all the time. As was pointed out by Etheredge, Jones, and Lewin (1996: 94) in a seminal article on what is propelling health-system change, "the percentage of workers in private firms who are enrolled in some form of managed care grew from 29 percent in 1988 to 70 percent in 1995." Moreover, economist Robert Kuttner (1999: 664) reported that "in the case of HMOs, the proportion of members who were enrolled in investor-owned health plans increased from 42 percent in 1987 to 62 percent in 1997." To provide a full understanding of the implications of this new pattern, I need to document what these changes have meant for the profession of medicine. Then I will take a look at how physician autonomy has been reduced and physician discontent has been on the rise.

Cost containment of health services has replaced benefits as the key concept in the minds of private and public purchasers. Less-is-more thinking has encouraged competition among insurers and providers to gain access to "covered lives." Premiums for employers under straight indemnity principles were always based on experience rating, a way insurers set the price for the following contract year. The idea of private insurance payers paying for an open-ended set of fee-for-service health insurance benefits has given way to one of defined contributions. With managed care plans, contributions are also augmented by greater responsibility on the part of the insured, both in paying the premium and in co-payment requirements.

As a result, purchasers and consumers have had to take a longer look at what their health care dollar will buy. Defined contributions also means that benefits officers seek out what is affordable to the firm. Purchasers seek deep discounts from providers and will accept "good enough" care rather than optimal care. In mature markets, where two or three major health plans cover 75 percent of covered lives, the insurers dictate the terms and conditions of contract to anxious providers (Kuttner, 1999: 666).

Still, if consumers want something beyond the "plain vanilla" product, they are going to have to pay extra. Purchasers, in the labor-scarce growth economy of the roaring nineties, were forced to bend to the wishes of employees demanding choice. By 1996, according to the American Association of Health Plans (AAHP), the lobby for the managed care industry, 92 percent of workers were offered at least one plan that covered out-of-network providers. At the same time, nearly 10 percent of employers provided undiscounted indemnity health coverage, down from 70 percent in 1988 (Kaiser Family Foundation and Hospital Research and Education Trust, 1999).

Employers have also required that employees shoulder more of the premium costs and established bigger co-payment requirements for seeing plan doctors and for using the plan's prescription coverage. Co-payment requirements not only shift costs to consumers, but also discourage utilization, as has been found in numerous comparative studies on physician visits when no co-payments are involved versus those with co-payments. Significantly, although 64 percent of Americans have employer-sponsored coverage, as many as 9 million uninsured Americans who are eligible for employee-sponsored health insurance have elected not to take it. As the American Association of Health Plans (AAHP) report on the individual choice model of health insurance noted in March 2000, "this decline in the 'take-up' rate is often attributed to the increase in employees share of insurance premiums" (p. 5). With the average employee share of premiums in 1999 approximately $35 per month for individual coverage and $145 for family coverage, employees in low-paying jobs have to make a careful and painful financial decision as to whether they can "take up" the offer of health coverage (Thorpe and Florence, 1999).

For more affluent American workers in the end of the last and the beginning of the new century, choice of provider remains more important than low-cost premiums and the absence of co-payments. The preferred-provider organization model (PPO) has swept ahead of the health maintenance organization (HMO) as the plan of choice among purchasers. AAHP figures show that 54 million people joined PPOs between 1991 and 1996, whereas HMOs signed up just 29 million. The average cost per member, per year is slightly higher in PPOs than HMOs, according to 1998 data. Point-of-Service plans are more expensive than either of these options, and employee enrollment in PPOs is now close to 100 million (Dalzell, 1999).

In the oversupplied, and consequently, fiercely competitive world of health-care providers, managed care plans can use their economic muscle to leverage price discounts. Specialists' fees were falling before the turn of the century like the value of technology stocks in the spring of 2000. "As managed care takes hold, providers' expectations have shifted toward a future of unrelenting pressures on pricing for downsizing" (Etheredge, Jones, and Lewin, 1996: 97). Moreover, the natural partnership between doctors and hospitals, so successful under the fee-for-service system, is riven by concerns about provider incomes, as health plans seek to squeeze even more slack out of the health care system. Hospital/physician alliances may break apart as their interests no longer are mutually supportive.

The day when the physician was completely in charge of patient-care decision making is gone. The use of practice guidelines, derived from studies of clinical effectiveness, although not accepted by many physicians, are used in managed care organizations at an increasing rate. The day when specialists were held in higher esteem than generalists may be gone since prevention and early intervention have become the signature activities of managed care plans. And the day when clinicians took pride and communicated to the populace that they were excellent in dealing with life-threatening and debilitating diseases has given way to concerns that medical groups and managed care plans do not want to attract patients who are expensive to take care of. Attracting good risks and avoiding bad ones have become the marching orders of the day, an essential survival technique.

Self-employment among doctors may also be endangered. A major trend has been toward physicians becoming salaried, usually in physician-owned group practices, and the predictions are that this trend will increase during the twenty-first century (Gold, 1999: 14). By forming groups, physicians seek to use their numbers to receive better contracts from HMOs and PPOs. In the past, the only salaried physicians were those who worked directly for staffed HMOs, academic medical centers, or medical colleges. Most doctors and physician-owned medical groups are now seeking contracts with several health plans at the same time. Every year, about one in five physicians' practices experiences extensive changes such as a merger, affiliation, or acquisition. Although change may be good for integrating health care delivery systems, there are winners and losers. Specialists have found themselves being turned down for participation in HMOs or PPOs as primary care providers begin to shoulder more of the load of patient care in the United States.

PHYSICIAN INCOME DECLINES

The reversals of fortune experienced by specialists and generalists under managed care is a story that also reaches into the academic side of medicine, revealing current and future income patterns. Medical students are shifting their career goals toward primary care and away from subspecialties where they are likely to see fewer patients and receive discounted fees. Medical school debt remains a constant burden for residents and other trainees at academic medical centers and hospitals nationwide, no matter what career option is selected. The fill rates in residencies such as anesthesiology, pathology, and diagnostic radiology fell sharply in 1995 and 1996, whereas there was more competition for placements in primary care training programs (Simon and Born, 1996: 132).

The first evidence that the managed care environment was affecting physicians' incomes was reported in 1996 (Simon and Born). Physician income had risen steadily at a rate of 5.9 percent, from 1982, the first year current income statistics were collected, through 1993. But physician income dropped 4 percent when 1993 results were compared with 1994. The largest reductions were experienced by those in the top 10 percent in earnings. Consistent with the market effect of managed care, specialty providers' income dropped far more than primary care providers. In metropolitan regions with high levels of managed care market penetration, incomes of physicians dropped more rapidly than in other regions, and incomes of owners of practices shrank more than those of salaried physicians, suggesting that they may be losing patients in the intense competition generated by managed care. In this market-driven health care environment, physicians may reluctantly accept capitation when joining an HMO panel or agreeing to substantial discounts to PPOs to gain access to covered lives.

Although payment through capitation increased during the 1990s, it was more likely to be found in large group practices than in small ones. Profitability under such contractual arrangements rests largely on restricting utilization, particularly referrals to specialists. Groups also reinsure against the possibility of large losses from catastrophic medical events when patients need extensive services. Although in some metropolitan regions, such as Boston, capitation is more prevalent than in others, discounted fee-for-service remains the dominant payment system under managed care (Simon and Emmons, 1997).

The decline in physician income has produced changes in physician behavior. Where in the past physicians provided charity care or reduced their fees for low-income patients, managed care has had a definite effect on discouraging this form of doctor largess. The uninsured and the underinsured should take note. A national study of 10,881 physicians, surveyed in sixty randomly selected communities, found that the number of hours of charity care provided in the month prior to the interview was sharply lower among respondents who derived at least 85 percent of their practice remuneration from managed care plans. Additionally, in areas with great market penetration of managed care, physicians who were not themselves strongly involved in managed care plans were less likely to give free care or reduce fees than in other areas. In total, 77.3 percent of the physicians surveyed provided an average of 10.3 hours of charity care per week (Cunningham, Grossman, St. Peter, and Lesser, 1999: 1087).

Financing has changed many aspects of our health care system. The social capital of the health care system in the days of fee-for-service medicine may have been exaggerated. Still, it was the foundation of cooperation, charity care, and cross-funding of worthwhile endeavors such as teaching and research. Whatever was there has given way to the social indifference of the marketplace.

PHYSICIAN SATISFACTION IN THE NEW AGE OF MANAGED CARE

I suspect the doctors who have given up charity care are not very happy about it. Charity care was a special act in a profession that honored social service, similar to the chef's signature dish in a great restaurant. As with the respected workman of the nineteenth century, American capitalism has taken on one of the most tightly organized professions and has, in the words of Karl Marx, stripped it of its halo. This reduction in status, income, and power was not predicted, even among the most keen analysts.

The attack on medicine came not from a rival occupation or profession, but from purchasers of health care.[1] As recently as 1986, the distinguished sociologist of professions Eliot Freidson said in *Professional Powers* that credentialing serves to create "an occupational cartel which gains and preserves monopolistic control over the supply of a good or service in order to enhance the income of its members by protecting them from competition by others" (p. 63). Even though the medical profession still credentials doctors through medical school education and hospital-based training, access to patients, or covered lives, has become subject to gatekeeping, more and more, by managed care organizations. It is the corporations, and to some extent the Center on Medicare and Medicaid Services—the wholesale purchasers of health care—that credential and control access to medical services for employees and their families, and Medicare and Medicaid recipients. By having a monopoly over the highly contested health care dollar in a market where suppliers are in surplus, the purchasers have broken the cartel.

How did individual physicians experience this transformation? To find out about physician experiences with managed care, the 1995 New York City–based Commonwealth Fund carried out a random, national cross-sectional survey of 1,368 office-based medical doctors who practice mainly in group or staff HMOs and have extensive contact with patients. Eliminated from the study were radiologists, pathologists, and anesthesiologists, physicians who have only fleeting or indirect patient contact. As the authors of this study, Collins, Schoen, and Sandman (1997: 2) reported in their introduction to their findings,

Questions covered physicians' level of participation in managed care and its effects on conditions of practice, clinical autonomy, ability to spend time with patients, and others matters. Physicians were also asked to characterize the type of plan in which most of their patients were enrolled, excluding patients insured under Medicare and Medicaid. As a result, the study includes comparisons across the various managed care arrangements now in use.

Given the ambitious scope of the study, the response rate was a dis-
appointing 48 percent, yet the authors suggested that time pressures in
the new financial and organizational world of managed care may have
created some incapacity to respond to a twenty-five-minute telephone
interview. More than 40 percent of respondents answered two questions
about managed care scheduling during the past three years by saying
that they have less time to spend with patients or with their colleagues.
Managed care has also added to the administrative burden of practicing
medicine, particularly in solo practices. More income declines than increases were mentioned, and specialists were the most likely to report
declining remuneration, mostly because of discounted fee-for-service
payments.

Adding to the changes produced by this new environment, 38 percent
of those who were interviewed said that over the past three years their
ability to make decisions that they think are appropriate for their patients
had diminished. "Almost a fifth (18%) are somewhat or very dissatisfied
with their authority to make right decisions, and nearly a third (29%)
say they are dissatisfied with the amount of time available for patient
care" (Collins, Schoen, and Sandman, 1997: 3).

Sixty percent of physicians sampled said that external reviews and
limitations on their clinical decisions were interfering with their practice
of medicine. Clinical autonomy was also reduced, according to four out
of five respondents, by the need to stay abreast of ever-changing insurance plan practice guidelines and utilization rules. The more plans physicians participate in, the greater the level of dissatisfaction with their
ability to make the right decisions for their patients. Only one out of four
physicians interviewed was satisfied with the practice of medicine overall. Physicians practicing in group or staff HMOs were more likely to be
satisfied with their practice than others, although they were more likely
to feel time pressures than doctors in other types of practice settings.

Disruption of practices through the loss of patients was correlated with
the high penetration of managed care in some metropolitan areas. Physicians also reported high levels of turnover. One of five physicians surveyed reported a voluntary or involuntary departure from a health plan.
Movement in and out of health plans means having to unlearn and re-
learn new practice guidelines and bureaucratic procedures, including the
conditions under which referrals are made.

Once, access to consultations with specialists was almost automatic.
HMOs that use primary care physicians as gatekeepers were reported in
the interviews to provide incentives to encourage these generalists *not*
to make referrals. In addition, where referrals were called for, between
23 and 31 percent of physicians said their attempts at referrals were
denied by their health plans. In contrast, "among physicians in traditional fee-for-service plans, nearly two-thirds say they have encountered

no serious problems in referring to specialists of their own choice, and 57 percent have had no serious problems with reviews of clinical decisions prior to a patient receiving care" (Collins, Schoen, and Sandman, 1997: 4). To compensate, some patients have become expert in knowing what their rights are in given plans and challenge primary care providers when they are not allowed to see a specialist (Jauhar, 2000).

In another national physician survey conducted by the Center for Studying Health System Change, the results about physician satisfaction were more ambiguous than in the Commonwealth Fund survey. Seventy-six percent of physicians said they were not hampered in their efforts to provide the best care for their patients. Specialists (27%) were more likely to say they could not provide quality care when compared with generalists (18%) (Reed and St. Peter, 1997).

Whereas the Commonwealth Fund study excluded radiologists and other physicians who had limited patient contact, the American College of Radiology executed its own study of its members in a 1995 survey. Questionnaires were mailed to a stratified random sample of 3,024 diagnostic radiologists, radiation oncologists, and nuclear medicine specialists. The results provided by the 75 percent who responded indicated a decline in satisfaction. Only 51 percent of radiologists in the 1995 survey would recommend a career in radiology to a college-age adult, a drop of 14 percent from 1990. When asked if they enjoyed working in radiology more or less than five years ago, 41 percent said they liked it less, and 22 percent said they liked it more.

The picture of managed care supplied by the radiologists surveyed had more influence on their professional satisfaction than did its administrative burdens or the actual percentage of patients in managed care plans in their practice (Crewson and Sunshine, 1999: 589). To what extent are these levels of satisfaction declining?

A survey of Massachusetts primary care physicians conducted in 1986 and 1997 found a substantial decline over fifteen years. Although both samples said the levels of care provided met their professional expectations, there were declines over time in the respondents' satisfaction with most areas of practice, the time spent with patients, the amount of leisure time they had, and the incentives to provide high-quality care (Murray et al., 2001).

In addition, further data analysis found that the physicians who worked in practices that contracted with multiple insurers were the most likely to be dissatisfied. They also reported more insurance company denials than those who worked exclusively with one health plan. Moreover, fewer than half the doctors interviewed said they would recommend these plans to family members or friends (Murray et al., 2001).

To what extent does such dissatisfaction lead to physicians migrating frequently from plan to plan? Are there disadvantages for patients when

their plans have high rates of turnover among participating practitioners? Are patients aware of provider dissatisfaction? To what extent are
physicians aware of these new pitfalls in medical practice?

Physicians need to learn how their profession operates within the new
system. Perhaps they also need to become more knowledgeable about
how to deal with the increasing managerial domination and decreasing
professional focus of contemporary American health care. Two sociologists, Castellani and Wear (2000), did qualitative interviews with fifty
practicing physicians. Many of the respondents felt utterly lost in this
brave new world of health care. Predictably, and painfully, the subjects
of this study felt unprepared for the struggle to balance concerns about
cost and patient welfare. Just as medical students need to be educated
about how practice is shaped by the new market forces in health care,
the veterans of the golden age and the new era of attrition need to get
smarter in the way of large organizations. In addition, the medical profession needs to regain its focus on the commitments that won the respect
of the public when state licensing was a goal.

Professionalism and professionalization require a new foundation in
medicine. Castellani and Wear (2000: 504) suggest that a social movement may be emerging in medicine:

Physicians need new ways to critically and self-reflexively think about the new
corporate health care systems in which they work and find ways to integrate
cost with care, ethics with economics and professional commitment with bureaucratic expectation.

In no specialty in medicine is this more evident that in psychiatry and
mental health services.

THE BATTLEGROUND OF BEHAVIORAL HEALTH

The most angry physicians today are found in psychiatry. Managed
care organizations have been most involved in cost cutting when dealing
with the treatment of mental illness. Even some primary care physicians
have complained that they are having difficulty making referrals for
mental health services. With approximately half of all practicing psychiatrists participating in at least one managed care contract, the need to
receive approval for hospital admissions by psychiatrists or extending
therapy sessions becomes much more of a concern among the members
of this specialty group. Utilization requirements, a form of cost control
that often limits practitioners' ability to provide the best care possible
for their patients, are part of the concern. In addition, psychiatrists object
to the use of treatment guidelines for managed care plan enrollees. In

the language of a group from Johns Hopkins (Domino, Salkever, Zarin, and Pincus, 1998: 149),

These guidelines serve as selection criteria to help determine not only which members of the insured population receive treatment for mental health care, but also to determine the allocation of enrollees to staff members and to prescribe the starting point for the types of services received.

Often health plans will not allow psychiatrists to do anything more than medication management for patients, with some consultation permitted to psychologists and social workers who are performing psychotherapy. Using the less expensive provider has become the signature of behavioral health care.

"Behavioral health care" is used to refer to a discrete organization of the delivery of mental health services that managed care organizations contract for with a provider organization. The emphasis is on cost containment through intensive case management and capitated payment for the entire basket of services used. It is based on rationing of services, so to accomplish this goal of cost containment, providers agree to do only what the behavioral health organization designates as medically necessary and at discounted rates.

Mental health services have long been a particular target of rationing, despite evidence that mental health services represent only about 8 percent of all revenues spent on health care annually in the United States. Because there was a perception among benefits managers that employees were abusing their mental health benefits, often in collusion with their mental health providers, managed mental health care was originally touted as a way to cut costs (Saeman, 1997). Two specific areas where utilization was disproportionately high, inpatient psychiatric and adolescent care, allowed attention to be drawn to this health-care sector, providing a screen on which to project concerns about costs. These services become "the ripest target" for scrutiny since it often appeared that no care coordination was taking place (Anders, 1996). At the same time, well-publicized scandals in the for-profit mental health services sector in the 1980s, particularly in Texas, revealed lengthy stays that were medically unnecessary, and fueled an effort to deny care (Iglehart, 1996).

Concern about costs was abetted by a cultural movement to "debunk" psychology, often considered by conservative public intellectuals and talk show hosts as a handmaiden of the welfare state. Many of those who now denied the efficacy of psychotherapy jumped on the bandwagon. Debates about whether or not psychotherapy "works" became popular; providing psychotropic drugs rather than therapy became a way to cut costs (Rothbaum et al., 1998). Concerns about quality and ethics fell by the wayside. Restricting access to mental health care helped cut costs (Anders, 1996). Offsets in other costs (for example, days lost from work) produced by clinical mental health interventions were ignored. A joke circulating in New Jersey in 1997 sardonically said that an accurate advertisement for managed care, including managed mental health care, would be, "Congratulations! You have chosen the cheapest plan with the poorest benefits."

Professional opinion against restrictions on benefits was manifest *before* the invention of behavioral health management service provider organizations. The logic of discharges under behavioral health management services appears to be equivalent to betting against the house in a Las Vegas casino—a no win. If the patient shows signs of improvement, the insurance reviewer may insist on discharge; if the patient is making no progress, the reviewer may still insist on discharge on the basis of the premise that the treatment is merely custodial (Gabbard et al., 1991: 319).

Critics of managed care applications to psychiatric treatment offer anecdotal information that suggests that the reviewers were trained in Alice in Wonderland logic rather than in psychiatry. Gabbard and his associates (1991: 318–23) analyzed managed care a decade ago from a psychodynamic perspective. In essence, they assessed the clinical effect of managed-care review. They noted that this form of disease management created uncertainty for the already vulnerable patient who was making progress—but not in a straight line. Following an analysis of the borderline personality, these clinicians suggest through detailed case material that there are serious consequences for patients who have difficulty processing this information; moreover, treatment team members have difficulties working with a patient when they know that treatment time is limited; and families of patients are affected as well when given a different view of the need for treatment by the reviewer. In sum, expectations of closing opportunities can create a sense of panic.

Managed care's inroads in psychiatric treatment did not stem from rising costs alone. There has always been some bias in medicine against psychiatry, but even medical doctors know that there are real diseases that affect mental states and make people dangerous to themselves or others, or create real suffering in people who cannot fully take care of themselves.

There are some valid studies that demonstrate the importance of outpatient psychiatric treatment. Summarized by Leon Eisenberg in the April 16, 1992, issue of the *New England Journal of Medicine*, these studies show how depression can lead to more days lost from work than chronic conditions such as hypertension, diabetes, advanced coronary artery disease, angina pectoris, arthritis, back problems, lung problems, and gastrointestinal disorders. Depressed patients identified by a structured telephone diagnostic interview were worse off than medical patients in 17 of 24 comparisons. In a second study, based on a community-derived sample, the number of days bedridden for a sample of 3,000 patients was 4.5 times greater among those with a major depression than in asymptomatic people. And the risk in people with minor depression was 1.5 times that in asymptomatic people.

In sum, these studies indicate that disability days frequently occur for people with psychiatric symptoms and that appropriate treatment is needed. Not only is this humane, but it also makes good economic sense since this treatment can reduce the use of other medical and surgical care. Psychosocial care needs to be viewed as a serious benefit, not a frill. How can this be done? Three basic principles guide the construction of any behavioral health care program.

First, behavioral health providers of direct care and primary care providers need to communicate frequently and work in partnership rather than as adversaries. Newly proposed federal law and existing state statutes, give the hospital and medical benefits for the treatment of mental illness parity with the benefits for treatment of physical illness. Under parity laws—the same coverage as for general medical services—insurers cannot limit the number of days they pay for mental hospital stays to less than those that will pay for other kinds of hospital admissions. Nor can plans impose arbitrary limits on out-patient mental-health services. Most health plans have an upper limit on the number of days of hospitalization they will pay for in a given year.

This may serve to reduce stinting when it comes to interventions for emotional or thought disorders. A study of states that have parity laws has shown that there are no increases in premiums for employers who provide health benefits to employees, especially when they introduce managed behavioral health programs (Zuvekas et al., 2002). Violations of these new laws may generate lawsuits against insurers or employers who fail to furnish equal treatment for all those covered, no matter what the disease. In addition, cost cutting may be counterproductive since evidence exists that counseling services for workers reduces the number of days lost through sickness or absenteeism.

Second, preventive intervention could reduce stress. And stress avoidance is often learned by patients during counseling or therapy. In managed care, teaching patients to give up smoking or curtail alcohol intake is considered a good way to reduce the need for more intensive kinds of care in later life, for example for stroke, heart disease, or kidney failure.

Finally, psychiatric treatment can be accountable to insurance carriers. Utilization review is the form of peer accountability that has been generated by the American Psychiatric Association (APA), to assure that necessary and appropriate care is delivered. The APA developed peer review services in the early 1970s to furnish insurers with the option of offering psychiatric care, limited only by medical necessity. This system has enabled insurers to achieve savings through cost avoidance in other areas of medical care. Psychiatrists review each case, working within guidelines established by the APA's *Manual of Psychiatric Peer Review*. Documentation of savings has been demonstrated with private insurers Aetna and Mutual of Omaha, and with CHAMPUS, the federal government's insurance program for dependents of military personnel.

With these three principles in mind, an appropriate benefits package can be created that includes psychiatric care that allows healing time for serious cases and cuts down on the negative consequences of the failure to treat.

Predictably, the limits on their practice with managed care patients also becomes a source of dissatisfaction for psychiatrists. Psychiatrists' experience served as the opening round in the struggle to contain costs by limiting the physicians' autonomy. The former editor of the *New England Journal of Medicine* Jerome P. Kassirer once wrote (1994: 634) about the golden age of medicine:

Once upon a time doctors had nearly complete professional autonomy. If they completed their training, and were certified by a professional board, they were assured the respect and trust of the public, and virtually no one kept track of their professional performance. What a difference a few decades make!

Despite this rueful remark, the more fundamental question remains whether and how physicians can serve as patient advocates in a cost-driven environment. The trends in the rapid growth of the PPO, largely based on discounted fees (and the slowdown in membership in HMOs), may have been one response to a backlash among professionals and consumers to the limits on the clinical autonomy of physicians. With physicians required to see more patients to make up for giving discounts, professional dissatisfaction may increase as physicians have less time for diagnostics and to interview patients with medical problems. We have come full circle ethically: from unnecessary care and wasting scarce resources and sometimes putting a patient at risk, to not giving necessary care and carefully husbanding scarce resources. Some partisan observers of the current medical scene have called for medical schools and graduate programs "to make students and trainees more aware of the conflict between traditional professional values and the imperatives of the market so they will be better prepared to defend these values in the new business climate" (Relman, 1999: 463).

And what about practicing physicians? According to Castellani and Wear (2000), some physicians are actively becoming sophisticated about corporate health care and its forms of organization. How will their professional and personal commitments fit within this system that is a work in progress? More important, to what extent will the rules and regulations of managed care interfere with the basic trust that must be established between doctor and patient? Marc Rodwin (1995: 605) raises some of the legal and ethical issues relating to who should protect the patient from lack of information. "If managed-care organizations do not fully disclose their policies of limiting services, should physicians as fiduciaries also inform patients of medical options that managed-care organizations exclude?"

And should doctors inform patients of their own financial incentives to reduce services? Perhaps a new medical ethics needs to be generated. In Chapter 6, I explore some of these efforts at creating a new code of ethics for the organizational restraints on autonomy in the managed care era.

American medicine gained its power, prestige, and privilege riding the small business model of service delivery. All the clinically practicing members of the profession mastered the same medical school curriculum and had graduate training as clinicians with technical knowledge of their fields. The organizations in which they worked allowed individual autonomy, subject to peer review of a gentle and nonintrusive kind. Collegiality allowed physicians to feel they were participating in a community of practitioners if not a community of scholars. Even when external review criteria were imposed, the observations were minimal and the sanctions were minor.

To bring American medicine into the twenty-first century requires going beyond the highly individualized form of professional autonomy to which the doctors who took care of me as a child in the 1940s and 1950s adhered. Doctors are being herded into group practices, giving them the opportunity to learn and improve as they get to see the best of their peers at work. At the same time, they should take advantage of the opportunity to become involved in joining teams to engage in multidisciplinary problem solving.

On the financing side, doctors and their patients must demand that quality be rewarded. Keeping down expenses is not as important as keeping people well and promoting wellness among those with serious chronic illnesses. Incentives that promote teamwork and quality care could become the hallmark of managed care. In the words of Kenneth I. Shine, president of the Institute of Medicine,

Payment methods must provide fair payment for good management of the type of patient seen, and there must be a way for providers to share the benefits. The experience has been that incentives are important, but we need to align them and provide an opportunity for consumers and purchasers to recognize quality differences and then make decisions accordingly. Payment systems should align financial incentives to the implementation of care practices based on best practices and on the reduction of fragmentation of care. Systems demonstrating this ought to be rewarded. (2002: 94)

The centralized incorporation of health care and its vertical integration have made the work of doctoring very different, even when technical advancements in diagnostics and treatment has made medical interventions more decisive than in the past. We need to explore that new corporate world and the partnering and contracting that has become the new way in which health care is organized and delivered.

Yes indeed, a quip is in order: Is Dr. Seymour Patients in the house?

NOTE

1. Eliot Krause did point to the death of the professions as we know them, but did not predict the rapidity of the transformation of the American health care system.

REFERENCES

American Association of Health Plans (AAHP). 2000. *Individual Choice Model of Health Insurance* 1 (March). Washington, DC: AAHP.

Anders, G. 1996. *Health against Wealth: HMO's and the Breakdown of Medical Trust.* New York: Houghton Mifflin.

Bauman, P. 1976. "The formulation and evolution of the health maintenance organization policy." *Social Science and Medicine* (April/May): 129–42.

Colby, D.C. 1997. "Perspective: Doctors and their discontents." *Health Affairs 16* (November/December): 112–14.

Pope, G.C., and Schneider, J.E. 1992. "Trends in physician income." *Health Affairs 11* (Spring): 181–93.

Castellani, B., and Wear, D. 2000. "Physicians views on practicing professionalism in the corporate age." *Qualitative Health Research 10* (4) (July): 490–506.

Collins, K.S., Schoen, C., and Sandman, D.R. 1997. "The Commonwealth Fund survey of physician experiences with managed care." Available online at http://www.cmwf.org/programs/health_care/physrvy.asp.

Crewson, P.E., and Sunshine, J.H. 1999. "Professional satisfaction of U.S. radiologists during a period of uncertainty." *Radiology 213* (2) (November): 589–97.

Cunningham, P.J., Grossman, J.M., St. Peter, R.F., and Lesser, C.S. 1999. "Managed care and physician provisions of charity care." *Journal of the American Medical Association 281* (March 24/31): 1087–92.

Dalzell, M.D. 1999. "With PPO enrollment nearing 100 million, HMOs are getting a health dose of competition. Is the PPO here to stay—or just a temporary distraction?" *Managed Care* (June): 1-8.

Domino, M.E., Salkever, D.S., Zarin, D.A., and Pincus, H.A. 1998. "The impact of managed care on psychiatry." *Administration Policy in Mental Health 26* (2) (November): 149–57.

Eisenberg, L. 1991. "Treating depression and anxiety in primary care: Closing the gap between knowledge and practice." *New England Journal of Medicine* 326 (April 16, 1992): 1080–83.

Etheredge, L., Jones, S.B., and Lewin, L. 1996. "What is driving health system change?" *Health Affairs* 15 (Winter): 93–104.

Freidson, E. 1986. *Professional Powers.* Chicago: University of Chicago Press.

Gabbard, G.O., Takahashi, T., Davidson, J., Bauman-Bork, M., and K. Ensroth. 1991. "A Psychodynamic perspective on the clinical impact of insurance review." *American Journal of Psychiatry* 148 (3) (March): 318–23.

Gold, M. 1999. "The changing US health care system: Challenges for responsible public policy." *Milbank Quarterly* 77 (1): 3–37.

Iglehart, J.A. 1996. "Health policy report: Managed Care and Mental Health." *New England Journal of Medicine* 334 (January 11): 131–35.

Jauhar, S. 2000. "Even doctor-patient relationships can be dysfunctional." *New York Times* (April 25): F7.

Kaiser Family Foundation and Hospital Research and Education Trust. 1999. *Employer Health Benefits 1999. Annual Survey.* Oakland, CA: Kaiser Family Foundation and Hospital Research and Education Trust.

Kassirer, J.P. 1994. "The use and abuse of practice profiles." *New England Journal of Medicine* 330 (March 9): 634–36.

Kuttner, R. 1999. "The American health care system: Wall Street and health care." *New England Journal of Medicine* 340 (8) (February 25): 664–68.

Mechanic, D., and Schlesinger, M. 1996. "The impact of managed care on patients' trust in medical care and their physicians." *Journal of the American Medical Association* 275 (June 5): 1693–97.

Murray, A., Montgomery, J., Chang, H. et al. 2001. "Doctor discontent: A comparison of physician satisfaction in different delivery system settings, 1986 and 1997." *Journal of General Internal Medicine* 15: 451–59.

Perkins, B.B. 1998. "Economic organization of medicine and the Committee on the Cost of Medical Care." *American Journal of Public Health* 88 (11) (November): 1721–26.

Reed, M.C., and St. Peter, R.F. 1997. "Satisfaction and quality: Patient and physician perspectives." *Data Bulletin Number 3: Results from the Community Tracking Study.* Washington, DC: Center for Studying Health System Change.

Relman, A. 1996. "What went wrong with the Clinton Health Plan." A review of Theda Skocpol, *Boomerang: Clinton's Health Security Effort and the Turn Against Government in Politics*, 1995, New York: Norton. *New England Journal of Medicine* 335 (August): 601–2.

———. 1999. "Education to defend professional values in the new corporate age." *Academic Medicine* 74 (5) (May): 463–64.

Rodwin, M.A. 1995. "Conflicts in managed care." *New England Journal of Medicine* 332 (March 2): 604–7.

Rosenbaum, S., Frankford, D.M., Moore, B., and Borzi, P. 1999. "Sounding Board: Who should determine when health care is medically necessary." *New England Journal of Medicine* 340 (January 21): 229–32.

Rothbaum, P.A., Bernstein, D.M., Haller, O., Phelps, R., and Kohout, J. 1998.

"New Jersey psychologists' report on managed mental health care." *Professional Psychology: Research and Practice 29*: 37–42.

Saeman, H. 1997. "Wall Street, more than managed care, responsible for health care changes, former psychiatry president declares." *National Psychologist* (September/October): 18, 20.

Shine, K.I. 2001. "2001 Robert H. Ebert Memorial Lecture—Health care quality and how to achieve it." *Academic Medicine 77* (1) (January): 91–99.

Simon, C.J., and Born, P.H. 1996. "Physician earnings in changed managed care environment." *Health Affairs 15* (3) (Fall): 124–39.

Simon, C.J., and Emmons, D.W. 1997. "Physician earnings at risk: An examination of capitated contracts." *Health Affairs 16* (3) (May/June): 120–26.

Thorpe, K., and Florence, C. 1999. "Why are workers uninsured? Employer-sponsored health insurance in 1997." *Health Affairs 18* (2) (March/April): 213–18.

U.S. Department of Labor 1996. *A Look at Employers' Cost of Providing Health Benefits*. (July). Washington, DC: Department of Labor.

Zuvekas, S. H., Regier, D. A., Rae, D. S., Rupp, A. and Narrow, W. E. 2002. "The impacts of mental health parity and managed care in one large employer group." *Health Affairs 21* (3) (May/June): 148-59.

4

The Reorganization of Health Care Delivery

How do managed care organizations (MCOs) become successful? The principle that operates in putting together providers and patients is to pass along deflation. Indeed, if inflation is passed on in the way wages chase prices, then deflation is passed on in a race to see who can do it the most cheaply. It is a race to the bottom—and that is precisely what worries providers and patients. Can quality of and access to care be maintained if resources are conserved?

As with any organization that creates some output or changes the environment in some way, the greater the integration of work facilities, the greater the productivity of each unit. MCOs are integrated organizations in the two ways that this concept is used in the literature of organizations.

Horizontal integration means that providers with the same skills and interests join together to create a group of great capacity to see large volumes of patients. Administrative costs per unit of service decline when this form of organization takes place. Economies of scale enter into the picture, reducing the costs of such support services as payroll, human resources, and telephone systems, to name only a few of the important services found in large organizations. More specific to health care, the group practice aspect of this form of integration allows expensive equipment to be shared among many providers, making technology, such as a magnetic resonance imaging machine, less expensive to maintain when it is used more hours a day than when fewer physicians make use of it.

In addition, a number of orthopedists can share ambulatory surgical units.

Where feasible, support staff can serve several providers at the same time, as when one receptionist answers the phone for ten doctors, makes appointments, and orders lunch. Similarly, one office manager can supervise the clerical staff and also make sure that medical supplies are on hand for physicians. When services are truly high volume, a number of simple medical tasks (for example, taking blood pressure) can be bundled and turned over to a nurse, a nurse practitioner, or a physician's assistant, freeing physicians to do complex assessments. Sometimes primary-care physicians are replaced with nurse practitioners not only as the first point of contact but also for the treatment of minor illnesses.

With a large provider network MCOs are better able to sell their services to benefits officers and other buyers because they can demonstrate a wide variety of choice among providers who agree to accept their discounted fees. In addition, the purchasing power of providers increases when the needed resources are bought in extremely large amounts. Selling will discount more for the big buyer than for the small buyer.

Vertical integration refers to the extent to which the highly differentiated providers and units work closely together, but performing the functions each does best. Management seeks to avoid inefficiencies such as duplication of services and use of expensive providers when less expensive providers can be just as effective, and employs decision making that promotes the kind of care wherein patients get exactly what they need and no more. Hospitals and physicians are sometimes linked together through financial arrangements so that there is mutual interest in seeing each succeed. Matters of clinical care then become the more closely shared responsibilities of these two parties. To make these decisions work, a refined continuum of care can also be established, including ambulatory surgery, home health care, skilled nursing care, and hospice care. Coordination of care makes it possible to fit the patient to the needed service rather than provide a single service, which may be the only type of care available.

This modern form of integration is built on models created more than twenty-five years ago. Pulling together a large number of physicians, hospitals, and other facilities was once the dream of health planners in the 1970s as a way of dealing with the uneven development of services. What this model suggested was that services should be distributed according to need. A given city, suburb, or metropolitan region might have far too many doctors and hospitals in proportion to its population, whereas some other locations might be underserved. Planning the distribution of primary-care services—small local, district hospitals for secondary care, large regional hospitals for tertiary care (for example, open-heart surgery), and a university medical center for teaching and training—would create the right access for the entire population. Regionalization of this kind of care would mean that a network of services would be available for every 2 to 3 million people (Roemer, 1973).

Some of the nonprofit health maintenance organizations (HMOs), such as Kaiser-Permanente, started to create organized delivery systems during the same decade in which health planners called for more rational distribution of resources. When they began to provide health care for a large number of people in the same locality, it became possible to create shared diagnostic and other services used by large numbers of providers. Having a great number of "covered lives" creates both adequate revenue sources and the need to plan services and promote coordination between units.

The logic of growth in contemporary MCOs starts with similar assumptions. The first step in being a successful MCO today is to get a contract with employers who can deliver a large number of lives to cover. This requires being willing to offer deep discounts to attract customers. Benefits officers are usually seeking to beat the national average expenditures for both MCO coverage and traditional indemnity insurance coverage. Because there is a great deal of competition among the MCOs in metropolitan areas, the corporations are finding that it is a buyer's market.

Still, these plans have to be attractive to employees and their families. Because employers often offer employees a menu of several options, MCOs need an assist from the employer to get employees to sign up. This assist usually comes from lower out-of-pocket costs for each family, both from lower deductions than indemnity coverage from the weekly or monthly paycheck and lower co-payments and no deductibles. This can be a powerful incentive, especially when wages and salaries are stagnant. Similarly, some corporations encourage their employees to enroll in the lowest-cost plan by picking-up a greater percentage of the total charges by the health plan than in the more expensive alternatives; saving money is another way of increasing a family's purchasing power.

Despite these incentives, some families are still reluctant to leave indemnity insurance that provides access to an esteemed provider. Patients with young children or with serious medical problems will often be loyal to their physicians. MCOs also learned throughout the 1990s that potential enrollees are discouraged when their own primary-care doctor or specialist is not listed in a plan's stable of providers. To encourage recruitment, MCOs often attempt to bring into their network the local doctors near a company that can give them many enrollees. It is of particular use to sign up a large number of pediatricians known to the employees.

Maintaining those relationships is important to parents. If those familiar and well-known providers are on the plan's list, then the decision to join becomes an easy one. When an enrollee has access to the same doctor at less cost, how can one refuse to enroll?

There is yet another inducement for joining the plan. A point-of-service option assures the enrollees that any doctor who accepts indemnity insurance will be available to them if they cannot find what they want within the network. Of course, they must pay some substantial first-dollar or deductible costs and usually also a 20 percent co-payment for every visit until some large amount of out-of-pocket expenses have been incurred.

This kind of option—a safety feature for those who are concerned about being locked into a panel of doctors—is not used that much, but it is reassuring to know that some insurance coverage is available if some recondite problem cannot be managed within the HMO's arsenal of providers. It can also be said that the point-of-service feature helps convert members into believers. This backup indemnity insurance provides a bridge back to trusted providers who may not join the network. If an HMO enrollee is in the middle of treatment with a non-network provider, that treatment can continue while the rest of the family takes advantage of the care available within the network. This is a clever way of creating confidence in a new and untried system of health-care delivery.

Similarly, the employer who signs on with one MCO may not be guaranteed the same price for a new contract in the future. Usually, when a purchasing decision must be made, a quick study is conducted of the indemnity insurance, or other MCOs' selling price, and a rapid calculation determines how much to charge the employers. The price quoted will usually be lower than the price quoted for indemnity insurance, but it will be close to that quote. The business pages of the daily newspaper refer to this as "shadow pricing." Sometimes rates are cut dramatically when a large number of subscribers sign on in one fell swoop.

The reorganization of the delivery system has been fueled by the use of capital accumulated by the large American health insurance corporations. Cigna of Connecticut was once a straight indemnity insurance company but rapidly reorganized itself into one of the largest vendors of managed care plans. Financial analyst and reporter Peter Kerr observes that this company is organizing a medical network that will dominate health care in the twenty-first century.

Since 1984, Cigna has organized about 150 networks that together serve more than 2.6 million people nationwide. The company will not say how much it has invested in managed care. But after years of losses its managed-care operations are now profitable and health plans are responsible for the lion's share of the company's earnings. (Kerr, 1993, Section 3: 6)

Increasingly, HMOs and other managed care plans like Cigna, by driving out or buying out weaker competition, have created mature markets in metropolitan areas, wherein five or six very large plans dominate the market share. Plans may acquire medical practices and other elements of a delivery system in an area where they do a great deal of business. In some parts of the United States, consumers and providers have widely accepted the HMO model. Gains in integrating services, as well as changing styles of medical practice, were noted in California at the beginning of the last decade. The result has been less use of diagnostic testing and referral to specialists (Freudenheim, 1991).

Sometimes, this kind of alignment becomes a liability. In Minneapolis, home of some of the largest HMOs in the country, employers started to reexamine the HMOs with which they had contracts, seeking not just savings, but quality. These giant corporations are starting to negotiate directly with medical groups and hospitals in the metropolitan area of the Twin Cities to promote new approaches to care (Winslow, 1995). One such provider network, Health Systems Minnesota, posted a doctor full time on a rotating basis at its participating hospital. Data on more than 400 patients showed that the presence of this physician in the wards shortened hospital stays and substantially reduced specialty consultations, thereby cutting overall costs per admission by 20 percent. Patients were pleased with the care they received, even though they did not get treated and monitored by their own doctors.

The battle for market share can also mean that HMO profits may be limited as charges to employers are kept low. With earnings down, companies whose stock is traded publicly may find that the price of their shares in the stock market decline. Other factors have to do with unpredicted changes in physician-practice styles related to prescribing or to hospitalizing patients, therein creating greater costs for the for-profits than were anticipated when they offered a proposal to corporations to become one of their health plans (Freudenheim, 1996).

LEARNING TO SAY NO

In the past, doctors were encouraged to do more for the patient for financial reasons and, to some extent, for fear of losing patients who perceived that their complaints required attention. Today, the incentives are reversed in managed care plans and providers need to convince patients that less is more. What this means is that they need to justify their medical decisions to skeptical patients who often feel they are being ignored because MCOs do better as an enterprise when they are cost conscious.

The physician payment system has certainly shifted away from the traditional fee-for-service format to include capitated payment and salary. After moving away from fee-for-service payment, consumer demand for direct access to specialists, skipping gate-keeping primary-care providers, has generated a new menu of ways of paying the doctor. In fact, hybrid payment systems exist. A doctor may be partly paid by capitation and partly by fee-for-service within the same plan. Is there evidence from comparative studies that shows conclusively that the payment system by itself leads to either unnecessary visits or stinting on services?

An invitational conference in September 2000 organized and operated by the Robert Wood Johnson Foundation sought to bring together diverse experts to review the literature on the power of payment incentives on physician behavior. Senior health plan representatives, physicians, and physician group leaders, state and federal policy makers, and health service researchers explored and deliberated on the subject of physician compensation for two days. Their conclusions were that much needed to be done to fully understand the effect of payment on physician behavior.

Not surprisingly, the major conclusion of conference participants was that effects of various payment structures on physician behavior, and ultimately on the cost and quality of health care, remains unclear. The degree of experimentation with payment structures in the private sector, however, suggests that how physicians are paid affects how they practice medicine. Although the current research on the effects of capitation versus fee-for-service is inconclusive, the meeting participants generally agreed that well-designed studies or demonstrations could shed some light on the effects of current payment structures (Health Care Financing and Organization: News and Progress, December 2000: 1).

The stories that doctors and health service researchers tell about how fee-for-service payment incentives lead to the provision of inappropriate and unnecessary services, or that capitation rewards the holding back on the delivery of appropriate services, did not find backing in the research literature. Even a straight salary was considered by health economist James C. Robinson as suspect: "salary undermines productivity and fosters a bureaucratic mentality of lack of responsibility among physicians" (Health Care Financing and Organization, December, 2000: 2).

Although physicians express largely negative responses to managed care and capitation payment because of the increased financial risks for providers and the micromanaging of their practices, there is little to show that patients are the losers. The conference participants found minimal support for the idea that physicians change their medical practice styles according to the way they are paid by a patient's managed care plan. Moreover, the complexity of the blended forms of payment discourages any unchallenged conclusions. The experts did conclude that practice styles were changing and that physician autonomy was under the knife, with some states more reorganized than others.

Again in California, we find a living laboratory concerning how managed care is transforming the delivery of services. James C. Robinson has been the chronicler of changing health care organization in the most populated state in the union. In a 1996 article, he reported on how HMOs affected hospital capacity and utilization between 1983 and 1993. Using multivariate analysis, he studied private nonprofit and for-profit hospitals with twenty-five or more beds in the Golden State. He found that HMO market penetration accelerated the substitution of outpatient for inpatient surgery and the shift from acute to subacute inpatient days and reduced psychiatric hospitalization.

Managed care has pushed the acute-care hospital from the core to the periphery of the delivery system. This change did not happen without guidance from experts on health outcomes. Not surprisingly, some companies create standards for clinical practice, telling doctors what to treat and how much treatment to provide. In addition, corporations such as the fifty-year-old firm Milliman and Robertson consult with the for-profit and nonprofit HMOs, advising them on what to cover and what not to cover. Needless to say, many doctors treat these guidelines as irrelevant to good medical practice because they regard each patient as unique. The American Medical Association, which has not produced its own guidelines, has fought the Milliman guidelines as unnecessary. Still, the AMA appears to be covering all bases: There is a report that the AMA is interested in buying the company as a way to set standards under its aegis.

The standards are set through extensive reviews of the medical literature and the study of medical records or charts to determine what works and what does not. The Milliman guidelines cover hospital admission and stays, office treatments, home health care, and recovery times for individuals before returning to work. Additional volumes in the future will address medication issues and dental treatments.

Run by the iconoclastic Dr. Richard L. Doyle, Milliman and Robertson depended on nine doctors to determine what they considered unnecessary hospital days. Since hospital per diem costs averaged $1,500 by the mid-1990s, the savings to health plans from reducing stays can be quite substantial. Throughout the country, use of these guidelines has reduced the number of days patients stay by one-third, particularly in California and the Midwest. The East Coast physician groups have resisted the use of length-of-stay guidelines and have sought to introduce legal challenges to their application in medical decision making (Meyerson, 1995).

The use of clinical treatment guidelines is only one way HMOs keep doctors from providing care that may get to be expensive and, at least according to these standards, not very effective. HMOs also attempt to manage physician behavior by recruiting and selecting only those physicians who can work under these kinds of restrictions. Any health delivery structure—or conditions that create uniform patterns of behavior—

requires selection and training so that management can get physicians who can work under rules. This means that younger, rather than older, physicians will be recruited since they are less likely to be set in their ways. A strong reliance on primary-care physicians, particularly those with training in family practice medicine, means that they will employ providers who are less prone to test, hospitalize, and refer to specialists.

A 1994 national telephone survey of 108 managed care plans described the different kinds of arrangements made with physicians according to the type of provider organization established (Gold et al., 1995). Recruitment standards varied, with the group or staff models having more demanding requirements than are found in independent practice associations (IPAs) or preferred-provider organizations (PPOs). Once accepted, turnover rates are low in all models of organizing physicians.

According to the Gold study, most HMOs require primary-care providers and specialists to go through a certification procedure. This procedure can "deselect" or weed out those with histories that predict they won't be cooperative or those who have been dropped from the practitioner rolls of other health plans. Then, physicians need to learn how to work under new financial incentives.

Among the network or IPA HMOs, 84 percent had some sharing of risk with primary care physicians, 56 percent used capitation as a primary method of payment, and 28 percent used fee-for-service payments in some form along withholding or bonuses (p. 1680).

IPAs were most likely to use consumer satisfaction information to determine bonus payments, whereas group and staff HMOs rewarded productivity and tenure. Practice and utilization management were generally guided by policy, peer review, and outcome studies.

More than 95 percent of the HMOs and 62 percent of the PPOs had a written quality-assurance plan, a quality-assurance committee, and a patient-grievance system. Seventy-nine percent of the group or staff HMOs and 70 percent of the network or IPA HMOs required outcome studies for particular clinical conditions, had targeted quality improvement initiatives, and used outcome studies to identify needs for improvement and to gauge success (p. 1681).

The most recent form of organizing physicians is through independent and integrated medical groups. Clearly, this type of arrangement allows physicians to establish greater bargaining power with HMOs. In this way, doctors have attempted to resist the market pressures of HMOs by organizing into their own networks as well as seeking legislation to protect their rights or to limit financial incentives that encourage cost containment. Large medical groups in California have contracted with HMOs through capitation to provide integrated medical services on a per-member per-month basis. Each group is financially at risk for the costs of care. As Robinson and Casalino report, "These groups manage the full spectrum of care, including the services provided by their own physicians and those provided by outside physicians, hospitals, and ancillary organizations" (1995: 1684). Such medical groups compensate physicians through a fixed salary, with bonuses determined by physician productivity, patient satisfaction, and group profitability. And because they own their own hospitals, they can receive HMO payments for hospital as well as professional services.

Independent and integrated groups were successful in keeping the rate of hospitalization and patient visits well below the national average for HMO patients as well as for non-HMO patients. Most important, Robinson and Casalino were able to show that management techniques made a difference in cost containment.

Medical directors and physician committees at these California groups performed their own reviews of utilization and its management rather than hire consulting firms to perform these tasks. Using clinical information, this approach is cooperative rather than adversarial. Most important, it takes management functions out of the hands of the HMOs and allows doctors to review and reward doctors, eliminating the individualized negotiations that go on between HMOs and physicians in most state plans.

In the past, when doctors colluded to agree on what price to charge, the Federal Trade Commission often saw this practice as price-fixing, a clear violation of federal antitrust law. New rulings from the commission suggest that when it is deemed to be in the public or consumer interest for these combinations to occur, such arrangements will be viewed as encouraging competition, as when doctors combine to sell their services directly to an employer, thereby eliminating HMOs as the broker, and thus will be considered legal (Pear, 1996).

Under antitrust law, physicians could create a provider network only if they also assumed financial risk. Under the new rulings of the Justice Department, doctors could be paid on a fee-for-service basis, and the benefit for consumers would be in the form of better services through competition. By pooling information on prices and costs, provider networks would be in a better position to determine price setting.

The reorganization of services is also influenced by the new rivers of green, that is, money, in the field of health care. Cash infusions have promoted some new concentrations of provider control, or better, attempts to control providers. Strong financing by venture capitalists of new kinds of health-delivery organizations led to the sale of medical practices by physicians to practice management companies. The rapid accumulation of physician practices was slowed substantially when managers realized that the acquisition of a practice did not necessarily mean that physicians altered the way they used tests, performed procedures, and referred to subspecialists (Dudley, 2001: 1089).

Moreover, physician groups, some on the verge of bankruptcy, most recently have given up capitation contracts with major MCOs such as Blue Cross and Aetna. The doctors who run these groups are willing to take their chances that they can secure better arrangements on a discounted fee-for-service basis (Dudley, 2001: 1089).

DISEASE MANAGEMENT CARVE-OUTS

HMOs not only contract with existing integrated medical systems but also contract on a capitation basis with highly specialized provider systems that concentrate on delivery of services to people with specific diseases or behavioral problems. Under a "carve-out" arrangement, these contractors agree to assume all financial risk for the care of a particular population whose care the provider network or a staffed HMO considers very expensive. A capitation charge for the entire panel of "covered lives" generates the payment to the specialized provider program. From the HMO's perspective, this shedding of tasks allows management to lock in costs for the coming year, helping to make expenditures more predictable. This enables them to offer contracts that will be less likely to lose money through miscalculation of costs.

An HMO may contract with a company to provide all mental health services, ranging from psychiatric hospitalization, to outpatient therapy, and even to testing children suspected of having developmental delays. All management and delivery of these behavioral-health services, as they are called, are in the hands of the specialized provider. As shown in Chapter 3, some of these mental health service policies and practices are controversial because of the limits imposed on hospital days for psychiatric patients, who may need more time to recover, or because family may regard these patients as dangerous to themselves or to others.

Not all "carve-outs" generated so much professional concern as behavioral health services. Still, other new forms of service delivery encouraged by managed care created turf battles and other kinds of concerns. Just before the end of the last century, HMOs contracted with a real upstart in the cancer treatment field, a company run by Dr. Bernard Salick. This physician is applying the principles he learned in running dialysis units and his experience in getting care for his daughter who had bone cancer as a six-year-old. Starting on the West Coast, where many innovations in the United States have emerged, Salick has moved into large-volume cancer markets in Florida and New York City. His seven-day-a-week, 24-hours-a-day treatment services make maximum use of facilities, thereby driving down the cost of service delivery to each patient. Because his operation has high volume, he can also contract for deep discounts from pharmaceutical manufacturers and other suppliers (Rosenthal, 1996).

As you might have guessed, not everyone was happy with this innovative program. Cities with well-established programs that provide services and train oncologists were deeply threatened by the loss of revenues once the HMOs chose to turn to Salick Health Care to care for those with catastrophic illness. Moreover, Salick lured away some top specialists to direct these centers, start-ups linked to prominent hospitals that had little treatment capacity in this area before his arrival. Hospices lose referrals because Salick also offers palliative care as part of a comprehensive package to HMOs.

Analysts of the new forms of HMOs suggest that the real advances in managed care management come from responding to the two major components of the system: the providers and the consumers. As with any complex organization, there are internal and external markets that must be satisfied and controlled at the same time.

Providers need to learn to work within a system that downplays heroic intervention, an attribute physicians acquire during medical education and training. They need to make good decisions based on the limited resources they have available and their knowledge of what works and what is ineffective. This information must be kept continuously fresh to achieve the best outcomes. If the age of big government is over, so is the age of overtreatment and lack of concern for cost. Plans may need to do some medical "unlearning" as well as training about the rules and regulations of being a participating provider.

Good providers also need information about how well they are doing compared with their peers in order to maintain the goals and objectives of the commercial HMO-quality care at reasonable cost while still earning a profit. The nonprofits also need to learn how to use information effectively to improve care coordination and to determine whether the desired results are being achieved.

Data is also useful in determining the price of the health plan an HMO will sell in the marketplace. Consumers will be more receptive when they are given some choice of plans, perhaps available at the same seller. Plans should not consider "one size fits all," since American consumers look for choice even when distinctions between products may be minimal.

The business practices of HMOs and their collaborators helped reduce the rise of health-care costs in the 1990s during President Clinton's first term in office. Physician income declined in 1994, with specialists taking a 5 percent reduction. HMOs clearly have had the upper hand in bargaining, and even those physicians who do not participate in managed care plans have had to keep their fees down to avoid losing patients to HMOs.

Yet experts and the general public remain unconvinced that this market-driven transformation has led to better quality or a more satisfied consumer, despite the lack of convincing evidence that a significant de-cline in quality has occurred. Physicians Elwood and Lundberg, two major observers of our current health system, assert that quality im-provements will come about only when three conditions are met. First, there must be

strong national standards that hold these plans accountable for the results they achieve—either in terms of clinical quality, improving the health of their enrolled population, or even satisfying the expectations of their enrollees . . . Second, then purchasers and consumers will be able to reward or punish plans based on qual-ity. And third, when purchasers and consumers have . . . The tools that allowed them to buy on quality, and if they could actually begin to use that power to shape the market. (1996: 5)

In response to the way for-profit managed care plans have shifted control from the provider to the purchaser and the payer for services, physician groups and hospitals have sought to create alliances and part-nerships rather than own outright the resources they need to deliver services. These linkages reduce long-term commitments in constantly shifting markets.

California, once again, leads the country in undertaking these orga-nizational transformations. It is especially evident that when capitation is the major form of payment, and organized groups of doctors bear the financial risks, that integrated medical groups and IPAs, a network-form of physician organization with administrative supports but without own-ership or the need for much professional interaction, create new forms of organization. There is less desire to own needed service delivery sys-tems and greater interest in contracting to gain what is needed. Robinson and Casalino (1996), through use of in-depth interviews with the creators of these new organizational forms, have identified what they call "virtual integration."

Using a fixed amount of dollars effectively, these medical groups are built around primary care providers and engage in contracts selectively with specialist physician panels and hospitals. Another advantage of this form of organization is that it creates a medium for innovation. Robinson and Casalino (1996: 13) posit that "the medical group provides the or-ganizational context within which to develop a culture that promotes quality and cost-consciousness through internal peer review, combining economic efficiency with a culture of professionalism."

Most important, an integrated delivery system can create social capital between the hospital and physicians. If you can achieve the arrange-ments described below without the baggage of having to support an overbedded institution, then you can develop the virtues of vertical in-tegration and avoid the burdens of ownership.

Cooperation between physicians and hospitals can encourage efficient use of services for hospitalized patients and a smooth transition to post-acute care. Integration can discourage the duplication of clinical services such as radiology and administrative services such as utilization management and discharge planning. Ideally, an integrated organization can function as a seamless system within which patients can move freely from outpatient to inpatient to subacute to home health services (Robinson and Casalino, 1996: 17).

In sum, a virtually integrated delivery system offsets the economic responsibility of the medical group for the hospital and can work outside some of the rules and regulations of the hospital. Community practice of medicine makes the hospital less critical as acute patient care becomes downsized. Home care has become more important since patients spend so little time in hospital care. Coordination becomes central to the delivery of quality care. Contracting becomes essential to providing care at reasonable cost. In a changing environment, capitation requires that the medical group or IPO avoid cost centers. Being locked into a vertically integrated system means that it is harder to change incentives and create innovative delivery systems.

With primary care capacity the single most important factor in the delivery system, all kinds of new arrangements are possible. In Atlantic Coast states, where older, established delivery systems still are organized around tertiary care, the approach is different from the for-profit MCO world of California. Some vertically integrated delivery systems initiated by academic medical centers have bet their ongoing viability as providers of complex medical services on the establishment of large numbers of primary care offices in the community. Serving as feeder locations, these outposts provide primary care for patients covered under managed care contracts and, when appropriate, will generate sufficient demand for specialty services. Patient flow remains central to the financial and professional viability of the academic medical center when managed care principles seek to keep patients out of hospitals.

Some academic medical centers have taken even more daring steps. Columbia-Presbyterian Medical Center, with the support of Oxford Health Plans and several other HMOs, set up a primary care office in midtown Manhattan in 1997, staffed by advanced-practice nurses, called Columbia-Presbyterian Advanced Practice Nurse Associates (CAPNA). Given that nurse practitioners spend more time with patients, particularly doing health promotion, the MCOs are pleased. Guiding patients through weight loss or smoking cessation programs will offset costs later in a patient's life. Although some physicians take issue with the limited diagnostic training of advance-practice nurses, each nurse practitioner works closely with a supervising primary care physician. Nurse practitioners have admitting rights at Columbia-Presbyterian Medical Center, but they have to notify the collaborating doctor within twenty-four hours after an admission, and they are not permitted to manage patient care in intensive care units (Brenna, 1997).

Although this innovative program is not without its critics, it has been subject to evaluation. Most important from the perspective of the parent institution, New York Presbyterian, a union of two medical centers that merged in the late 1990s, this outpost funnels patients with serious illnesses to specialists waiting nearby at the impressive tertiary care facilities along the East River and to the north along the Hudson.

The New York City metropolitan area is overdoctored and overbedded, but Gotham's dwellers are not alone in witnessing a major transformation in the major institutions that deliver health care in this country. In Chapter 5, we will take a closer look at the changes the managed care transition has wrought on the ground of our nation's academic health centers, from sea to shining sea.

REFERENCES

Brenna, S. 1997. "Is there a nurse in the house?" *New York* (October 7): 51–54.
Dudley, R.A. 2001. "Managed care in transition." *New England Journal of Medicine* 344 (14) (April 5): 1087–92.
Eisenberg, J.M. 1996. "What went wrong with the Clinton Health Plan." A review of Haynes Johnson and David Broder, *The System: The American Way of Politics at the Breaking Point, 1996. Boston, Little, Brown. New England Journal of Medicine* 335 (August): 602-4.
Elwood, P.M., and Lundberg, G.D. 1996. "Managed care: A work in progress." *Journal of the American Medical Association* (October 2): 1–9. Available online at http://www.ama.assn.og/ . . . ol_no_13ed6063x.htm.
Freudenheim, M. 1996. "HMOs are having trouble maintaining financial health." *New York Times* (June 19): D12.
Freudenheim, M. 1991. "In a stronghold for HMOs, one possible future emerges." *New York Times* (September 2): 1, 28.
Gold, M.R., Hurley, R., Lake, T., Ensor, T., and Berenson, R. 1995. "A national survey of the arrangements managed-care plans make with physicians." *New England Journal of Medicine* 333 (December 21): 1678–83.
Health Care Financing and Organization: News and Progress. 2000. "The power of physician payment: Designing incentives in the new era. HCFO meeting discusses effects of payment structures on physician behavior." *Health Care Financing and Organization: News and Progress*, December 2000: 1–4.
Kerr, P. 1993. "Betting the farm on managed care." *New York Times* (June 27): Section 3; 1, 6.
Kilborn, P.T. 1996. "Tucson HMO's may offer model for Medicare's future." *New York Times* (March 20): D1, D5.
Meyerson, A.R. 1995. "Helping health insurers say no." *New York Times* (March 20): D1, D5.

Pear, R. 1996. "U.S. issues guidelines to help doctors form health networks." *New York Times* (August 29): A22.

Robinson, J.C. 1996. "Decline in hospital utilization and cost inflation under managed care in California." *Journal of the American Medical Association 276* (October 2): 1060–64.

Robinson, J.C., and Casalino, L.P. 1995. "The growth of medical groups paid through capitation in California." *New England Journal of Medicine 333* (December 23): 1684–87.

Robinson, J.C., and Casalino, L.P. 1996. "Vertical integration and organizational networks in healthcare." *Health Affairs 15* (1) (Spring): 7–22.

Roemer, M.I. 1973. "An ideal health care system for America." In Anselm Strauss (ed.), *Where Medicine Fails*, pp. 77–93. New Brunswick, NJ: Transaction Books.

Rosenthal, E. 1996. "A pushy newcomer shakes up cancer treatment in New York." *New York Times* (September 8): 1, 44.

Winslow, R. 1995. "Employer group rethinks commitment to big HMOs." *Wall Street Journal* (July 2): B1, B4.

5

Managed Care and the Profession's Tarnished Jewel in the Crown—Academic Health Centers

Health care as we know it has undergone a transformation equivalent to the way the Republican-dominated Congress of 1994, with its "Contract with America," forced President Clinton to make good on his claims to seek welfare reform. The institution of public assistance will never be the same. The institutions that make up the American health care delivery system have suffered a similar blow. From reports dealing with the facts on the ground, the commercialization of health care has torn away the aura surrounding academic-based medicine and interfered with its financial health. Moreover, financial issues have made the leadership of these organizations concerned with competing for patients with local hospitals and community-based physician groups.

The chief executive officers of these complex centers for tertiary health care, which deal with the most serious and life-threatening conditions, have lost prestige as they struggle for market share. The quest to collect "covered lives," that is, patients with adequate insurance who will use it when they need it—and who will fill hospital beds—has become the name of the game. Let's take a closer look at this transformation of academic health centers as they have been forced to stray from their contributive mission in American society during the fat golden years of health care to becoming lean and mean scufflers, or in today's lingo, nimble corporations that can survive in a new competitive environment.

In the recent past, goodwill, combined with surpluses, was a terrific formula to doing well by doing good. Good deeds remained unpunished. The social capital that allowed for charity care, or uncompensated care, as the accounting departments of hospitals called it, may be all used up. Cross-funding of research is harder to justify. And the trainers of the next generation of physicians now have little time to volunteer to make sure that students and house staff get it right by learning from their mistakes. Increasingly, clinical care delivered by medical school faculty in their private practices becomes a major source of support for medical schools and academic health centers (Ludmerer, 1999). The deal that cut everyone some slack so that good deeds could be done—the social contract—has come undone.

The original Clinton Health Security Act called for a partnership between managed care organizations and what were designated as "Centers of Excellence," akin to the Morningstar mutual fund rating for important health care delivery programs. Centers of Excellence are elite institutions—academic health centers where the most medically complex services are found (locations for tertiary care). Centers of Excellence are known for attracting fiercely competitive graduating medical students eager to complete their residencies at programs where star medical performers work. This category also characterizes facilities where a patient with a poor prognosis is sent, or where subspecialists who are superior diagnosticians hang their shingles. Academic health centers also house specialized diagnostic and evaluation units or clinics (for example, dealing with neuromuscular disorders) and, more often than not, treatment centers for rare and sometimes costly conditions such as hemophilia.

Academic health centers, despite their prestige and reputations for being on the cutting edge of clinical research, have been particularly vulnerable during this new age of managed care. Few accommodations have been made for their complex and necessary mission. Concern was expressed before the managed-care market reform took place. The Clinton-led health care reform task force tried to plan for "managed competition," so that these institutions would not be eliminated in a "race to the bottom" to deliver services at the lowest price. In the vision of the planners, managed care organizations (MCOs) would seek services from these existing citadels rather than reconstruct them anew. Interestingly, the health care reform task force assembled by Senator Hillary Rodham Clinton, then first lady, and her staff did not include much representation from leaders of medical schools or chieftains of the academic health centers of the United States.

With the defeat of serious government-led health care reform in 1994, the well-capitalized growth of managed care has accelerated. Under managed care, the integration of services and restricted access to hospitals and specialty care has left fewer options for the directors of these centers of excellence. Some criticism is in order when it comes to academic health centers' failure to teach residents and medical students how to use resources more carefully. Such teaching might have led to a less expensive way of delivering care without adopting the micromanaging practices of managed care organizations.

From the point of view of the leadership at academic health centers, at best, managed care is not necessarily the enemy of excellence. However, few of these CEOs would argue that it is their friend. But if left on its own, managed care will destroy much that is good in its zeal to rein in the cost of health care. It has long been recognized that managed care does not stand alone: It needs to include the complex functions provided by academic health centers (AHC) because their functions are hard to replace from a knowledge-based system of care.

The growth of managed care has been deemed the main reason that the current inflation rate in health-care costs is far below the high rates of the 1980s. Although the rate of cost growth may be diminishing, the access problem for those without insurance remains. The drive for greater efficiency in health-care delivery by health maintenance organizations (HMOs) has not done much to extend coverage to the uninsured, except in states that reformed their Medicaid systems to include more of the uninsured (Oregon, Tennessee). Nor has managed care been regarded by consumers as producing better care at less cost. Employees and other managed care plan participants perceive managed care as a necessary compromise if they are to receive *any* employer-subsidized insurance. Studies that measure consumer satisfaction with health plans, while demonstrating satisfaction within the same range as levels for fee-for-service plans, often reflect respondents' concerns about whether the plan will be there for them if they have complex medical problems. Those members of plans with serious chronic illnesses are more critical of what the plans provided than those without such conditions.

Centers of Excellence, because they earn their reputations as tertiary care centers that deal with the most complex medical problems in the most sophisticated ways, are special. Academic health centers are, at the same time, multifunctional institutions. Many of the tasks of medicine involve the continuous rebuilding of infrastructure through the creation of new knowledge and the renewal of human capital by exposing trainees or residents to the most difficult cases. Furthermore, these practical citadels of high-technology health care have been often the sole source of care for those without insurance or capacity to pay, including the homeless, undocumented aliens, or the near-poor who cannot qualify for Medicaid. They have done it with funding coming largely from federal subsidies for graduate medical education and support for hospitals with needy patients, and indemnity insurance payments that generated a surplus for these nonprofit corporations. These important functions in our health care system are weakened by the penetration of markets by managed care organizations and their consequent reduction in referrals and demands for lower fees.

There are some good reasons to refuse to continue to support all the activities undertaken in academic health centers as well as some dangers in trying to contain the high costs of subspecialization. A case can be made that hospitals and academic health centers are partly responsible for the oversupply of subspecialists in the United States. Here again, the silence of the AHC physician leadership is noted. The overwhelming interest on the part of subspecialty-oriented medicine in training sub-specialists was understandable, even if the numbers trained are excessive. By receiving payment from the Medicare program to do graduate medical education, administrators were able to meet their medical service needs with trainees, thereby reducing their costs in delivery of both inpatient and ambulatory care. Subspecialty residents, upon completion of their training, then go forth into practice, seeking higher fees than lesser trained physicians and practicing a style of medicine heavily dependent on the use of technology (Barondess, 2000: 1300). The social reproduction of specialization has led to a disproportionate distribution of physicians who cannot or do not want to do primary care. No country in the new millennium needs so many specialists. There are two specialists for every one generalist. In other countries the ratio is reversed or one-to-one.

The growth of specialization was not completely grounded in the economic incentives related to higher fees for specialists. There was a knowledge base for these new fields and their advocates. Biomedical research blossomed after World War II, and new technologies emerged, and along with them new subspecialties with recently trained clinical fellows and former residents who sought to increase their skills by using what they knew.

As the control over hospital admissions and access to specialists shifted more and more into the hands of primary care physicians under contract with MCOs, the fate of the academic health center became more and more uncertain. Since excess capacity meant that revenues to maintain the AHC were threatened, AHC executives started to discover ways to compete with community hospitals for contracts with managed care organizations. To hard-bargaining managers of MCOs, it made little sense to pay more for a bed in a university-linked hospital than in another hospital that had been certified by the Joint Commission on Health Care Organizations. Kenneth Ludmerer (1999), a leading expert on medical education, has written about how cutthroat competition has left AHCs in a difficult position.

To attract patients from managed care organizations, academic health centers had to compete with community hospitals on the basis of price. This was no easy task. Because of education, research, charity care, and a mix of patients, the costs of teaching hospitals ran approximately 30 percent higher than those of community hospitals. Previously, third party payers were willing to accept higher bills from teaching hospitals to cross-subsidize these socially important activities. Now insurers were increasingly unwilling to do so, insisting instead on paying only for the cost of the hospital care actually incurred by their members. (p. 354)

MCOs could get away with paying only for their immediate needs because of the oversupply of providers. They do not wish to sustain future health care delivery by paying for research and training now. It should also be noted that Medicaid and Medicare payments have been capped by federal legislation, reducing incomes for hospitals even further.

Today, as part of AHCs, hospitals are increasingly dependent on contracts with HMOs for inpatient care. Consequently, there will be fewer budgetary resources to provide subspecialty training or supply charity care to the uninsured. To their credit, hospitals and medical centers delivered uncompensated care through surpluses derived from per diem payments generated by third-party and out-of-pocket payers. Despite the shift in the last decade to a prospective payment system for Medicare patients (and subsequently for those with commercial insurance), attempts were made to provide emergency care and hospital care for individuals without insurance. Congress also prevented hospitals receiving federal assistance from turning away patients who had no insurance and could not afford to pay for services from emergency departments. Moreover, hospitals with a disproportionate share of the burden of caring for the poor, the uninsured, and the elderly received subsidies through legislative funding provisions for Medicare and Medicaid.

OPPORTUNITIES FOR BEDSIDE TEACHING IN THE ERA OF MANAGED CARE

The methodology of managed care is built around using primary care as far as it can go, reducing the use of specialists likely to use expensive testing and to hospitalize patients, and limiting hospital admissions and lengthy stays. Under these constraints, teaching residents becomes more difficult. The business philosophy of MCOs says go the least expensive way, which leaves little opportunity for teaching and learning. Today, much of the patients' work-ups occurs prior to admission, making residents' discovery and acquisition of skills more difficult. Learning about differences among patients and how these differences can affect diagnosis is a subtlety that requires the chance to compare and contrast. The new system of breaking down tasks into preadmission, hospital stay, and postdischarge has left house staff—another name for interns and residents—with little opportunity for learning how to ask patients questions about their complaints. They need to learn about patients' feelings and failings, not just trust the tests.

Is there enough time to talk to patients? Those who work in academic medical centers think the luxury no longer exists. In November 1999, the *New York Times* ran a series of articles about doctors in training titled "New doctors step into a turbulent world." Following three interns (Post-Graduate Year One) at St. Luke's–Roosevelt Medical Center, reporters discovered that trainees now spend more time learning how to dial authorization numbers at the managed care plan than how to interact with patients.

Even a department chairperson is bewildered by the current system.

It's like good luck in knowing what I'm supposed to do—what phone number I call and what behavior I'm supposed to follow so everyone is ecstatically happy. If we admit someone and we didn't make the right phone call, it affects revenue. Many people don't have a medical card on them. They didn't plan on getting shot that day. (Kleinfield, 1999: 7)

Older physicians complain more than the younger ones. Yet the residents are not about to give up and start selling real estate. Older doctors, when not complaining, try to shut out the turbulence and teach medicine, avoiding discussions of managed care. Some doctors have less time to teach because they are busy supplementing their income from clinical sources by serving as expert witnesses or participating in studies for drug companies.

One thing that is not taking place in New York's academic medical centers is an education in how to work within a managed care framework. N.R. Kleinfield, the author of the last article in the *Times* series, says,

If insurers expected a teaching hospital like St. Luke's–Roosevelt to groom a generation of doctors willing to obey the managed-care mantra, that did not seem to be happening. In the course of their year, all three of the interns, while appreciating some of the waste excised from medicine, had become of a piece in their increasing resistance to cost pressures and managed care. (1999: B7)

Structural changes in how health care is delivered in the new age of managed care interfere with on-the-job learning. The give-and-take of the medical encounter is eclipsed by the need to economize. In fact, the patient-discharge planning process starts as soon as twenty-four hours after admission. The craft aspects of the role of the professional are neglected under such systems. From the residents' perspective, "They are deprived of much of the opportunity to follow the course of disease since patients would be so quickly discharged" (Ludmerer, 1999: 359).

The reduction in revenues for medical care also affects other functions. Clinical research in AHCs has been built in part on the capacity of scientists (who were also medical doctors) to have access to clinical revenues to fund research activities. In the days when costs were not major concerns, research projects could be initiated and conducted in a manner that buried the actual equipment and labor time in per diem costs. The fact that these costs could not be easily disaggregated, in an era before computer programs were available, was a way of avoiding questions of who should pay for what. The comfortable relationship between payers and providers meant that some procedures performed on patients (or specimens taken from them) helped advance medical knowledge rather than benefiting directly the patient being treated. Today, some patient-care services provided in hospitals may be regarded by MCOs as research-related and therefore not valid activities related to a hospital stay. The informal, unstated mutual support between teaching, clinical research, and patient care that worked to sustain health care as an institution is of no interest to the business-oriented managers of MCOs.

The race to the bottom line also interfered with opportunities for physicians to do research and teaching on a voluntary basis. With fees-for-service deeply discounted, it often takes a specialist based in the AHC five or more days to generate the amount of income that could be produced in four days of consultations in the past, which leaves less time for research. With the arrival of MCOs, the old assumptions no longer hold when it comes to sustaining clinical research. A new arrangement, perhaps a new partnership, needs to be created. However, it will take time to create this new compact.

Even with the National Institutes of Health's new commitment to clinical research, clinicians who do not obtain these grants will have to be co-opted to participating in protocols. Moreover, MCOs, rarely concerned about the future, may discourage cooperation because it will mean more overhead or administrative costs for them.

Just as there is now fear that research will suffer with this new payment mechanism and system of organizing medical work, there is also concern that medical training will suffer. Traditionally, attending physicians devoted a portion of their day on-site at hospitals and medical centers to teaching house staff (interns and residents) and/or medical students about some of the aspects of care and how to deal with patients. Now with some primary-care physicians (PCPs) working under a capitation mechanism, there is far less control over one's schedule than in the past. In HMOs with high PCP-to-patient ratios there is little flexibility in the workday, so little time remains to devote to teaching the next generation of physicians the finer points of care.

Specialists face a similar problem, although they may not be expected by contract to see as many patients per day. Again, the deep discounts from the standard fee demanded by HMOs from participating physicians in exchange for large numbers of referrals means that doctors need to do more to reach the same level of remuneration than they did prior to the advent of managed care. Although in the past, teaching in AHCs was often donated or pro bono labor, it was a valued and esteemed activity. There are serious concerns at these centers about how to make up for the shortfall in mentoring that once was assumed to come with the territory when a doctor received admitting privileges to a hospital.

The support of these activities was part of the "connective tissue" that held American society together. Plans for reforming health care, while grand in scope, always recognized these important functions of AHCs. Although never perfect, these institutions' efforts to survive through mergers are barometers of a new health care crisis. Quality, access, and cost—the trinity of problems that made single payer an option and created the Clintons' Health Security Act—are back on the national agenda. Current legislative proposals seek to ensure that quality and access are not eclipsed by cost considerations.

Consider what our society would look like without academic medicine. Health care would be dominated by a barracks capitalism mentality. The profit-seeking side of health care might rule out knowledge-seeking activities unless there was some payoff for owners. We need to invent a new policy that saves academic medicine. AHCs could be funded using a tax on health insurance or managed care organizations. Distribution of funds would take into account the overproduction of specialists from these programs and create incentives to limit their numbers. We need to make sure that our world-class medical care and concomitant research and training programs are available for all Americans—embedded in all delivery systems—and are not just a memory.

NEW FORMS OF MEDICAL ORGANIZATION AND CENTERS OF EXCELLENCE

The reorganization of health-care financing under managed care calls into question the capacity of specialty services to maintain the quality of care and ease of consumer access given the new demands of tightly knit delivery systems. Integrated Provider Associations (IPAs) are medical center/physician networks established in a particular region. They often become the delivery systems for a number of privately and publicly financed managed care organizations. Vertical integration is the *plat du jour*, and although the entrée is tough but nutritional, it may not be completely digestible. What is happening in the health care system is going to produce a bevy of case studies for master's in business administration programs.

How do we begin such a study? IPA leadership must undertake important decisions in the creation of a "full-service" system. Utilizing limited premium dollars, an IPA has to make distributions of resources precisely because under these new systems of financing, cross-subsidization will be less and less possible. Thus to make the product they sell to MCOs competitively priced, IPAs often extract discounts from practitioners and seek other, less costly solutions to medical care problems.

IPA decision makers must determine whether existing Centers of Excellence are affordable under these new constraints. Leaders must decide whether to invite into the IPA not only primary care providers (PCPs) but also highly specialized units at academic health centers, such as Centers of Excellence. These decisions are somewhat different from allowing "any willing provider" to participate in a network, or the subsequent step of credentialing PCPs, because of the complexity of the units being considered for integration into the IPA.

Through the use of a multidisciplinary approach, some programs that deliver specialized services to people with serious chronic illnesses and/or disabilities have developed high-quality services. They have evolved from specialty clinics held one day a week at a local hospital, where patients with a particular disease were seen by a few interested medical specialists, to major specialty centers drawing patients from a wide radius. These centers are currently financed mainly by third-party payments from private or public insurers; special government subsidies and training grants also help offset the high costs of multidisciplinary diagnostic and therapeutic services as well as clinical teaching.

Health policy analysts need to comprehend the conditions under which IPA leaders seek to obtain services such as diagnoses, evaluations, and therapies required by patients with serious chronic illness and/or disabilities, whether they are from individual providers or from existing regional Centers of Excellence. Also, given the complexity of these patients' needs, and the low prevalence of many of these conditions, which providers, nurses, PCPs, or specialists become the case managers/coordinators of this care? To what extent are care coordination skills transferable from disease to disease, or, alternatively, to be effective, must case managers develop skills related to specific groups of diseases, such as neurological disorders?

Additionally, how is medical training affected by decisions to follow the least expensive pathway to service delivery? To what extent will specialty programs have the opportunity to inform future or newly practicing physicians about the services they provide, and why does a multidisciplinary team approach benefit patients? Finally, is there public awareness and involvement in decisions about services that affect the quality of life of people with serious chronic diseases and/or disabilities?

To answer these questions, we need to examine how current changes in the financing and vertical and horizontal integration of health care affect the provision of coordinated, comprehensive diagnostic and therapeutic services for special needs populations, which were previously found only in Centers of Excellence. This objective could be accomplished through a synthesis of knowledge about how IPAs conceive of these services and deliver them, either through collaboration with Centers of Excellence or by some other means.

The New York City metropolitan region provides an excellent setting to look more closely at the consequences of integration of the health care system. Data on individual practitioners indicate that many belong to more than five managed care plans. By 1997, according to the Greater New York Hospital Association, 112 out of 125 area hospitals were part of nine multihospital systems. Most frequently found was a system that contained between 5 and 9 hospitals, comprising more than half the multihospital systems in the region.

Given this trend toward integration, 85 percent of the systems in the region sponsor a physician organization. Yet many of the system-affiliated physicians remain outside these physician organizations, perhaps because they are salaried employees of AHCs or other healthcare delivery organizations. We need to examine the consequences of these organizational developments at AHCs for future care: How do they and their units respond to the changing health-care environment? Are professional activities continued when referrals are reduced and/or funding of graduate medical education via Medicare allocations is reduced sharply? Who negotiates on their behalf with the newly formed health systems? What happens when Centers of Excellence become redefined from "profit centers" to "cost centers" because payers are reassigning risk to providers?

Additional data gathering should take place in metropolitan regions such as Miami, Minneapolis/St. Paul, and the San Francisco Bay area, where managed care has even greater market penetration than in the New York metropolitan region. The organization and delivery of health care is undergoing some really unusual arrangements. A new innovation in the Twin Cities area places faith in the marketplace to bring doctors and patients together. The Vivius MCO "enrolls employers and individual physicians, allowing the physicians to set their own capitated rates for office visits, and allowing consumers to shop for a panel of personal providers from among enrolled physicians" (Health Care Financing and Organization, December, 2000: 4).

Data could be collected through interviews with the principals of IPAs and Centers of Excellence that employ multidisciplinary teams, as well as interviews with consumers, and by examining administrative information from IPAs and Centers of Excellence. The following topics need to be covered: (1) how negotiations were initiated and conducted and with what results; (2) changes in the kinds of services delivered to special needs populations; and (3) the extent to which service delivery has been improved by organizational redesigns and/or technological enhancements introduced by managed care. In so doing, this type of study will permit planners and policy makers to determine whether high-quality care for special needs populations is maintained or sacrificed in an age where cost drives service delivery.

PROGRAMS THAT SERVE PEOPLE WITH DISABILITIES

During the past two decades, disability advocates often saw professional service providers as adversaries because they limited the self-determination capacity of people with disabilities. Today, with managed care dominating the private insurance market and the prospect of commercialized Medicaid managed care for the poor and individuals with disability waiting in the wings, family-professional alliances to protect access to needed resources may be a more appealing definition of empowerment. Current efforts to create that type of unity are beginning to emerge at academic medical centers. Once perceived as the enemy of empowerment by families of children with disabilities, centers are now spearheading the fight to save Medicaid as we know it.

Public funding through the federal-state formula for Medicaid led to payment for many services vital to an improved quality of life for people with disabilities. Many of the kinds of services so important to children and adults with developmental disabilities are defined as "collateral" or "ancillary" therapies, reimbursed by Medicaid and health insurance. As a result, these labels and payment mechanisms are remote from the concerns of state officials who focus primarily on preserving the infrastructure of public health and acute care in their localities. Advocates of public budget restraint may argue against the use of the Medicaid and Medicare systems to pay for so many therapeutic, residential, or support services, but no other options are currently available or likely to be offered in the future. The adoption of the *International Classification of Impairments, Disabilities and Handicaps*—2 system by health service providers, researchers, and policy makers would create a strong justification for financing interventions that could reduce reliance on traditional medical care.

VIEWS FROM SOME STAKEHOLDERS

The professionals who provide highly specialized health services to the disabled are most sensitive to the changing financial picture brought about by managed care.

Access to rehabilitation services is a major concern for people with disabilities. The providers of such care are most sensitive to the need to support inpatient rehabilitation, which often costs $1,000 a day and more. Cost-containing MCOs have a great deal at stake in keeping people out of this form of care.

To determine the effect of managed care on these highly specialized centers, Gerben DeJong of the National Rehabilitation Hospital Research Center conducted a telephone survey of rehabilitation providers in three health care markets characterized by high market penetration by MCOs. DeJong concluded that for providers attempting to limit damage and restore functioning for a patient, the in-hospital acute care units would be the location of choice. However, in many instances managed care payers bypass inpatient rehabilitation altogether. They approve rehabilitation services but in subacute care units only.

Given this trend, rehabilitation providers have linked up with larger health care systems to encourage referrals from acute-care hospitals. Cost cutting has called into question a valid and cherished way of developing a treatment plan—the interdisciplinary team approach—wherein each discipline or department arrives at a plan of care through weekly team meetings. The give-and-take of these discussions may no longer be of value when the hospital is no longer the foundation of the rehabilitation service delivery system.

With managed care, the fee-for-service and cost-based methods of rehabilitation payment are vanishing rapidly, but full case-rate capitation has yet to come to rehabilitation in any significant way. Most acute and subacute rehabilitation providers in the three markets studied are being paid on a fixed per diem basis, where length of stay is negotiated depending on patient status and progress (DeJong, 1996).

A life lesson can be drawn from the experiences of physicians struggling to deliver care to people with disabilities. How can we reconstruct the social contract that made the AHCs citadels where new providers learned their craft and where clinical research led to innovative practices that saved lives or improved the quality of life for Americans? We have some principles to guide us. Cost should not drive quality out of health care. (Or to restructure a recent aphorism: The good should not be an enemy of the perfect.) We need to convince decision makers that the interdisciplinary approach within medicine is essential for providing care for adults with spinal cord injuries or identifying the scope and types of problems early in the life of a child with developmental disabilities. In the former case, intervention usually results in greater independence, integration, and productivity. In the latter case, early identification, intervention, and the prevention of secondary disabilities is cost effective. Placing a child in programs—and reducing the adverse effect of medical conditions—pays off in the form of gaining a more productive member of society while reducing opportunity costs, an expression health economists use to refer to activities (e.g., employment) given up by other members of the family.

LOSING SOME OF THE MISSION OF ACADEMIC HEALTH CENTERS

Evidence is starting to accumulate that the impressions that observers had about the reduction in institutionally supported research at academic medical centers were correct. Faculty at 117 medical schools were surveyed to identify how their clinical research was supported. When institutionally funded research, as a percentage of direct costs of research for 2,336 faculty, was compared in metropolitan regions with different degrees of managed care market penetration, Weissman and his colleagues (1999: 1093) found an inverse relationship between the degree of competition and the level of institutional funding. The relative amounts of support were almost twice as high in the less competitive environments than in the most competitive environments. This outcome could not be accounted for by greater research activity in less competitive areas. In fact, the more competitive the market, the less likely there was ongoing faculty-supported research.

As managed care steadily wore away the resistance of physicians to participating in plans because they were afraid they would lose their patient panel, academic health centers, too, began to adopt business techniques derived from the world of managed care. Decrying these trends, defenders of the faith, such as Kenneth Ludmerer (1999), suggested that these elite institutions were turning into their opposites: "It became increasingly difficult to distinguish some academic health centers from the for-profit hospital chains and HMOs they so often criticized" (p. 365).

The three-legged stool that supported quality—research, teaching, and patient care—was losing two supports. This process of disequilibrium resulted from total concern with the bottom line in an age when hard decisions had to be made. Even patient care could be a loss center—if patients were too expensive to care for—given the severely-discounted reimbursements negotiated with managed care plans. Getting a reputation that a health center was good at caring for complex cases was the kiss-of-death. The irony was not lost among the subspecialists: Being good at what you do could be something of a curse, because you would attract the most expensive, as well as the medically neediest of patients. Could an academic health center and the attending staff offer to do only some of the care to optimize a patient's health? Could they argue that some components of their institutions had to be eliminated because they were too expensive to run? Eventually, the most strapped and beleaguered institutions had to recognize that without a mission they would have no profit margin.

Some of the leaders of the profession began to fight back, seeking a form of moral and cultural renewal. Arnold Relman, retired editor of the *New England Journal of Medicine*, among others, began to call for a new kind of professionalism.

REFERENCES

Barondess, J.A. 2000. "Specialization and the physician workforce: Drivers and determinants." *Journal of the American Medical Association 284* (10): 1299–301.

Biles, B., and Simon, L. 1996. "Academic health centers in an era of managed care." *Bulletin of the New York Academy of Medicine* (Winter supplement): 484–89.

DeJong, G. 1996. "Medical rehabilitation undergoing major shake-up in advanced managed care markets." *Bureau of National Affairs' Managed Care Reporter 2* (February): 138-41.

Donelan, K., Blendon, R.J., Hill, C.A., Hoffman, C., Rowland, D., Frankel, M., andAltman, D. 1996. "Whatever happened to the health insurance crisis in the United States? Voices from a national survey." *Journal of the American Medical Association 276* (October 23/30): 1346–50.

Health Care Financing and Organization: News and Progress. 2000. "The power of physician payment: Designing incentives in the new era. HCFO meeting discusses effects of payment structures on physician behavior." *Health Care Financing and Organization: News and Progress*, (December): 1–4.

Jensen, G.A., Morissey, M.A., Gaffney, S., and Liston, D.K. 1997. "The new dominance of managed care: Insurance trends in the 1990s." *Health Affairs* (January/February): 125–36.

Kleinfield, N.R. 1999. "After med school, the ABC's of insurance." *New York Times* (November 16): A1.

———. 1999. "With wariness and joy, the interns are reborn as residents." *New York Times* (November 17): B7.

Ludmerer, K.M. 1999. *Time to Heal: American Medical Education from the Turn of the Century to the Era of Managed Care.* New York: Oxford University Press.

Weissman, J.S., Saglam, D., Campbell, E.G., Causino, N., Blumenthal, D. 1999. "Market forces and unsponsored research in academic health centers." *Journal of the American Medical Association 281* (March 24/31): 1093–98.

6

Doctors Respond to the Dark Side of Managed Care

For the medical profession, managed care has meant a reversal of fortune. The world of work is far more socially and economically complex than it once was, whether in the big academic health center in the big city or the small medical group in the leafy suburb. Incomes are remaining flat or beginning to fall. The warnings of the 1970s and 1980s by observers went unheeded, and now, doctors face the dilemma of whom they owe their allegiance to: the patient or the payer.

"May you live in interesting times"—an ancient Chinese curse—is the equivalent of being exposed to the evil eye at birth. And some doctors feel that fortune is followed by misfortune. The portents were there. The golden age of medicine represented the fat years, perhaps to be followed, as in the biblical dream of Joseph, by the lean years.

The decline of the medical profession's status and power is as fascinating as medicine's rise to power. Yet it is a domestic tale. In my meetings with people from other countries, often as part of my wife's business travels, the subject of managed care is rarely mentioned when I let them know that I am a health policy analyst and a sociologist of medicine. Rather, they are most interested in how the United States could have more than 40 million Americans without insurance coverage of any kind. This baffles me, too, and I try to give my interlocutor a dynamic history of the organization and financing of health care in the United States. Needless to say, Europeans don't understand how the richest nation on earth and the leading military power, can fail to provide appropriate health care for all its citizens. Even the Australians wonder from down under.

I don't get the same questions in the United States. It's not hard to get a conversation going on managed care in the United States. The problem is that it's hard to stop the conversation. Both of the following encounters took place in Massachusetts, where managed care has made great inroads. I was in a Boston tavern (not Cheers) a few years ago, watching an NCAA basketball tournament game, when my professional identity was revealed to my fellow barmates. I then heard horror stories about high-handed treatment by health maintenance organization (HMO) administrators or too little time spent with the doctor. Fast-forward to a genteel camping trip to a wildlife refuge on an island off Cape Cod. Within our party, I encountered an orthopedic surgeon, a rabid Red Sox fan who practiced in Boston's Beth Israel-Deaconnes Hospital. We had a lengthy discussion of his problems with the various plans in which he participated. And even though he hated the fact that Roger Clemens was a Yankee, and I as a Yankee fan received some of the fallout on this issue, we had many hours of enlightening discussion on his experiences with managed care plans. He left me with a final directive: Find a cure for managed care.

Doctors are an interesting lot. They are noticeably great shop talkers. From the days in which they do their clinical clerkships, usually in the third or fourth year of medical school, and well into retirement, you can overhear them holding conversations about new treatments or how to avoid the adverse effects associated with a drug therapy. But not today. Medical financing and bureaucratization are now the main topics. Complaints about the heavily discounted fees they are forced to accept to be part of managed care plans are accompanied by horror stories about their hours on the phone struggling to gain approval for a procedure from a utilization review organization assigned that function by a plan. The sound of falling prices is heard throughout the land.

At the same time, physicians labor to hold on to their patients by any means necessary. To promote patient loyalty, doctors today stretch the truth to gain coverage for their patients. These efforts include reporting nonexistent symptoms, or the fabrication of medical findings to assist a patient in securing coverage for treatment or services. Changing the diagnosis in the direction of severity helps gain coverage or keep a patient from being sent home from the hospital too soon (Hilzenrath, 1998).

These lies are committed not only with the patient in mind. In a questionnaire sent randomly to doctors in eight cities by Victor G. Freeman and colleagues at the Georgetown University Medical Center, 64 percent of those in areas with strong HMO market penetration said, in response to a hypothetical question, that a physician should provide false documentation, if necessary, to get a health plan to pay for surgery to prevent gangrene of the foot. This compared with 46 percent of physicians in areas where these health plans had lesser market share (Hilzenrath, 1998). Discussion of these deceptive behaviors, or how to evade the system, now go on in medical school classes and among residents in academic medical centers. It may be viewed as the price of doing business rather than as a moral failing.

If lying *for* the patient goes on, what about lying *to* the patient about the optimal medical strategy to pursue versus what the managed care plan will pay for? Some managed care organizations (MCOs) have created "gag rules"—limits to what patients may be told about their treatment by plan-participating physicians. "Gag rules" restrict a physician's autonomy and are perceived as forbidding them from discussing therapeutic alternatives with patients that are not covered by managed care plans. Representatives of the American Association of Health Plans (AHHP), a national trade association, argue that these rules merely prevent doctors from saying disparaging things about the managed care plan and do not affect discussions of treatment options. After the dismissal of Dr. David Himmelstein, an outspoken critic of HMO policies and practices, from U.S. Healthcare's Boston Plan in 1995, a number of state lawmakers pushed to pass legislation to prevent "gag rule" clauses from being introduced in the contracts signed by physicians when they become part of managed care plan networks, a move generally backed by state medical associations.

To some extent, the health plans and their national association argue that patient trust is not needed since they have established a new evidence-based medicine in which doctors are more rigorously evaluated, screened, and reviewed than with the old "failed" fee-for-service system. Doctors are losing their charismatic roles in the face of death and disability and are being replaced by bureaucratic role performers who check off the boxes to indicate that they have done a thorough job. Is trust irrelevant under these conditions? Do restrictions on physician autonomy actually benefit patients?

Bradford Gray, a medical sociologist and health policy analyst, suggests that there will be efforts to replace trust in individual physicians and the profession in general by the generation of ethical standards and certifications in the managed care industry (1997). The promotion of the National Committee for Quality Assurance, by the American Association of Health Plans, is clearly one such effort. This nonprofit organization was established to reassure the public that the industry can police itself. Even greater trust is invoked by organizations in the nonprofit sector, such as the Foundation for Accountability, which reviews managed care practices independently and may help reassure the public that their welfare is being protected. The employment of doctors in executive positions within the industry suggests an effort to demonstrate that managed care is being led by people steeped in professional ethics, that the executives wear white doctors' coats.

No wonder Bodenheimer and Casalino (1999), in their intensive interviews with MCO medical directors, found that for these executives health care is simultaneously a profession and a business.

The medical director must work within a fixed budget and is accountable to the organization's chief executives who may not be physicians. . . . The chief medical officer acknowledges that he leads by persuasion, not by control. In one large national, for-profit HMO, each regional medical director reports both to the chief medical officer and to the regional manager. The highest-ranking person in each region is the manager, not the medical director. (p. 1946)

On another level, in national publications read by doctors, voices are raised that seek a revision of the ethics of medicine to deal with this new potential source of professional destabilization. Still other voices call for new forms of professionalism in medicine. In both cases, the theme is the same: The profession needs to be reformed to meet the current conditions on the ground.

One of the first attempts to raise the issue of the conflicting loyalty for the physician under managed care came from Marcia Angell in an article that appeared in an ethics journal titled "The doctor as double agent" (1993). Now the editor of the prestigious *New England Journal of Medicine*, Dr. Angell lamented the diminution of the fiduciary relationship with patients now that her peers worked both for their patients and their companies. Expected by patients to optimize their care, they were also expected—and rewarded—by their managed care plans to deliver those services at the least possible cost to the plan. Sociologists would call this a classic case of "role conflict," but an instance where eliminating one role, as a strategy for reducing tensions, would not be possible. The conflict was structured within the set of roles associated with one position. The doctor's dilemma could not be eliminated in modern America unless she retired or limited her private practice to those who paid out-of-pocket or with the rare indemnity policy. Much of the discussion that followed the publication of Angell's article focused on the need for a new professional ethic to respond to the managed care era.

REFORMING THE PROFESSION ON PAPER

The operant social construct in health care that many physicians perceive has shifted the concern from patient welfare to profits has been the increased privatization of the field. Once seen as a social service or public responsibility to be carried out without concern for market conditions, health care is now viewed as a private industry. In journals and other public venues, leaders in the profession have weighed in for more than a decade on the dangers of privatization to professional autonomy and patient welfare. Sounding like a contemporary of the youthful Karl Marx, Arnold Relman, editor emeritus of the *New England Journal of Medicine*, suggests that new relations of production dominate health care. Consequently, doctors now believe that

their ability to take appropriate care of their patients is being compromised by the cost management and the coverage decisions of insurance companies. Their own overhead expenses have risen as they struggle to survive in a new competitive and commercialized marketplace, and to comply with the red tape and the regulations generated by multiple payers. Reimbursement for their services is being capped or reduced, while increasing rewards go elsewhere in the system. (2000: 38)

Letters to the editor after recent news stories about physicians who cannot take care of their patients according to their standards point to the fact that doctors are being subject to enormous cross-pressures. These letters express enormous anguish and frustration (*New York Times*, 1999). Newspapers have the space to print only a few of the many letters they receive. Doctors don't just exchange information on how to best treat patients. They also complain about changes in the organization and financing of medicine.

These new social conditions surrounding medical practice cry out for a new professional ethical code, and some bioethicists have already started to create one. These fledgling efforts can be divided into the idealist and realist schools. Emanuel and Dubler (1995) develop the normative standard of the patient-physician relationship, a standard that may or may not be endangered by managed care. The Emanuel and Dubler model is composed of six components: choice, competence, communication, compassion, continuity, and (no) conflict of interest. Although they acknowledge that it is an ideal construct, the authors seek to use it to identify opportunities and threats generated by managed care to the patient-physician relationship, and to proffer ways to deal with such threats.

A few of the ethical statements that have been constructed for the brave new world of managed care begin with the hard reality of the day: Rationing services is necessary to keep spending on health-care services from continuing to take up more-and-more of the gross domestic product. The choice for the United States is to micromanage resources at the point of contact with the patient or to shift to a state-run allotment system, with each region getting a fixed sum to take care of its citizens' health needs. Some health policy analysts see rationing as the next big thing, as discussed in this statement.

> Rationing, defined broadly as resource allocation, is necessary and inevitable in some form, and bedside rationing (defined as individual physicians declining to administer beneficial treatments because of costs to someone other than the patient) is usually preferable to centralized, rule-based rationing. (Hall and Berenson, 1998: 396)

The ethical physician must start with this concern as well as the need to preserve the patient's trust that the provider will look out for his or her best interest. As the physician's role changes from the healer without limits to the protector of society's scarce resources, new ethical standards are required to guide its performance. Hall and Berenson note a paradox where patient trust is concerned: The more "at-risk" the patient, (that is, the closer to being in a life-endangered state because a decisive technology is not available), the greater the need for trust and the more the conditions for rationing prevail. They argue that financial incentives should influence but not determine physician behavior. Consider the following guideline they profess will help prevent possible rifts between patients and physicians (pp. 398–99):

- Physicians should not enter into incentive arrangements that they are embarrassed to describe accurately to their patients.
- Maintaining an ethical system depends on both consumers and professionals having the ability to exercise choice about whether to participate in a particular payment system.
- Physicians should be wary of incentive arrangements that are not in common use elsewhere in the market.
- Physicians should not steer their patients into different insurance plans according to the arrangements that will produce the most physician revenue: sick patients into fee-for-service, healthy ones into capitated plans.

As a defense against being guilty of patient disloyalty, the physician is encouraged to separate or distance herself from the medical restrictions of the plan, so long as a minimally appropriate medical response to the patient's needs is possible. Here, the presence of clinical-practice guidelines, a medical director who may make insurance coverage decisions, and the practice of peer review helps furnish support for a physician being denied authority to create a treatment plan.

Alternatively, the world of managed care has engineered the treatment of psychiatric disorders that involve little psychotherapy and a great deal of psychopharmacology. Brief office visits, in which an assessment of the patient's reaction to the medication is the main objective, and a quick check on progress or the lack of it, leaves no time to get to know the patient and teach her coping mechanisms to deal with life's stresses (Luhrmann, 2000). Such fleeting relationships leave the provider as lost as the patient and render both the patient and the provider little spiritual nourishment.

There is also an almost revivalist spirit being expressed in the major medical fora throughout the land. The essence of medical practice—an extreme dedication to serve society—is perceived as under threat. In manifesto-like style, Wynia and others (1999), three physicians and two attorneys, recall the spirited prose of yesteryear as they open their article in the *New England Journal of Medicine* on medical professionalism in society:

Today, at the dawn of a new century, a genuine medical professionalism is in peril. Increasingly, physicians encounter perverse financial incentives, fierce market competition, and the erosion of patients' trust, yet most physicians are ill equipped to deal with these threats. (p. 1611)

Starting at the beginning, this gang of five seeks to define professionalism as something that involves "both the distribution of a commodity and the fair allocation of a social good but that is uniquely defined according to moral relationships" (Wynia et al., 1999: 1611).

Professionalism is a form of social capital that needs to be saved and invested to protect vulnerable parts of the population. To rein in cutthroat competition and human indifference to the plight of those in need, the public's basic information needs and opportunities to establish protections against tyranny reside in professionalism as an institution (Wynia et al., 1999: 1611).

New advocates for professionalism identify these core elements:

• Devotion to medical service in the form of dedication to their craft even when financial rewards are below expectations.

• Resistance to financial incentives that put patient care at risk.

• Public profession of values that are shared with peers and that include acceptance of accountability for one's actions

• Negotiation regarding professional values and other social values, leading to a social contract.

When guided by these principles, professionalism will lead to activism in defense of vulnerable populations, such as the uninsured, or vulnerable institutions, such as academic medical centers even when doctors are not directly affected by these issues. Activism is on a continuum from patient advocacy and support for public health efforts, internal dissent from inappropriate policies in their managed care plans, and public dissent in the appropriate fora. Moreover, public dissent can lead to professional disobedience, as when professionals refuse to obey rules or laws that undermine good health care practices, and, if necessary, to a principled exit from medical practice.

This call for a restoration of professionalism in the face of the commodification, or the turning of health care into a marketable product, does not go far enough for some critics. David Rothman, a social historian and advocate of a public ethic for medicine with regard to such issues as the medical and pharmaceutical experimentation that takes place in underdeveloped countries, has suggested that managed care is basically a distraction from these far more important concerns (Rothman, 2000).

Some observers of the current scene wonder why doctors do not more publicly demand greater emphasis on quality and a return to professional autonomy. Margaret Mahony, M.D., (2000) suggests that physicians have a trained incapacity to speak out on issues related to patient care. She attributes this deficit to dehumanizing experiences in medical school and residency. Suffering in silence, doctors-in-training learn early on to hide their feelings.

Some doctors are not suffering in silence but are fighting back against managed care organizations' control over the practice of medicine. Like the hero of Ernest Hemingway's short story *To Have and to Have Not*, doctors are learning that a guy alone don't stand a chance. By 1995, a small number of physician groups were competing directly with MCOs by seeking to sell their services directly to employers (Freudenheim, 1995). And twenty-one state medical societies are assisting in the formation of physician networks.

There is some evidence that the elite institutions in American medicine have received a wake-up call. Advocacy for the preservation of the doctor-patient relationship is considered a requirement of medical practice today. Although everyone in the profession pays lip service to the need to promote businesslike efficiency, there is equal concern for putting the patient first. Dr. Bernard Lown, a Harvard cardiologist and co-recipient of the Nobel Peace Prize for organizing physicians against nuclear war, led a call for a moratorium on corporate takeovers of health services and for an end "to intrusion in the doctor's decision-making" (Kilborn, 1997, A12). This call to action was signed by many of the Harvard faculty and two-thirds of the 188-member graduating class of Harvard Medical School.

Petitions are being complemented by economic actions. Doctors in group practices, with the encouragement of the American Medical Association, are gaining business skills to permit them to eliminate the need to contract with the insurers.

Many group practices are acquiring the ability to largely duplicate the services generally provided by H.M.O.'s. They include eliminating wasteful practices, taking the financial risk of per capita contracts and rewarding physicians for keeping costs down. (Freudenheim, 1995: D7)

As reported in previous chapters, doctor discontent is widespread. With some doctors retiring early and others seeking nonclinical positions in medicine, there is clearly a desire to return to an earlier time. Jerome P. Kassirer (1998) reported that this wish is the father of the deed in a small number of cases.

A small, vocal minority of doctors have opted out of managed care contracts and accept as patients only those who are covered by indemnity insurance or who can pay directly out of pocket. Others, unhappy with the constraints of managed care, have moved to states in which managed-care penetration is (currently) minimal. (p. 1543)

How effective have physician associations been in responding to managed care? In a panel discussion sponsored by the Center for Studying Health Systems Change (1999), in Washington, D.C., a number of experts attempted to develop a framework for understanding physician and hospital organization in the era of managed care. The case studies that were discussed ranged from modest success in Boston to an "autopsy report" on medical centers in Phoenix and Tucson. The major conclusions drawn about the formation of successful management of physician organizations were the following:

- Physicians need to play central roles in all facets of the organization and should delegate those tasks in which they are not expert (p. 12).
- Physician organizations that accept risk and that are successful need to have physicians accountable to other physicians, especially in large groups where they do not all know each other (p. 12).
- Shared loyalties (i.e., social capital) between physician and hospitals remains important (p. 16).
- Information is important to these organizations, especially where capitation is the major form of remuneration to doctors, and it is capital-intensive, that is, expensive (p. 19).
- Risk adjustment payments may be necessary to prevent risk avoidance on the part of practitioners (p. 29).

David Blumenthal, M.D., was most eloquent when it came to justifying this last point, speaking about how a few transplant patients can be an enormous burden in a capitated practice; they also can be the source of professional satisfaction.

Without risk adjustment, those patients cannot survive in a capitated market. And the initial impression, the first impression that all of us had when we went at risk, or the first question we had was, are we going to have to give up what we all took most pleasure in as physicians, primary care physicians affiliated with an academic health center, and that is the ability and opportunity to take care of very sick outlier kinds of patients. (p. 29)

One of the unresolved problems of physician organizations is how to balance the needs and demands of doctors who take care of very sick patients against those who do not. Distributing funds is not an easy task in these newly formed organizations when capitation is squeezing all providers.

SUE THE BASTARDS!

Physicians do not like to sue because they are often the target of malpractice suits. They may even find the legal profession their enemy. However, when managed care plans fail to deliver what is promised, or when there appears to be uniformity in the approaches taken by MCOs, situations have become litigious.

In an unusual and unprecedented two-pronged attack, in early 2001, two groups representing 7,000 Connecticut physicians brought suit against six health maintenance organizations (Zielbauer, 2001: B1). The petitioners claimed that these large insurance companies arbitrarily denied needed medical treatment to patients and illegally withheld payments to doctors. The suit was filed in conjunction with the Nutmeg State's attorney general's office and was based on that state's Unfair Trade Practices Act.

This legal action was supported by the American Medical Association and was filed by the Connecticut State Medical Society. The society's six suits were aimed at stopping what it called " 'unfair, deceptive, improper practices' " that put patients at risk (Zielbauer, 2001: B8). In addition, five lawsuits were brought by a group of doctors who sought both to stop these practices, which were regarded as damaging to patient welfare, and to collect damages from insurance companies for failure to make legitimate payments to these physicians.

In April 2001, the National Healthcare Cost and Quality Association

(NHCQA) newsletter, an e-mail-linked Internet publication, reported that federal racketeering laws (RICO) were cited as being violated in four states by eight major health plans. Medical associations in California, Florida, Georgia, and Texas went to the courts to stop MCOs from exploiting physicians' services. Clearly, doctors are mad and they won't take it anymore.

GOING BACK TO BASICS—DOCTORS WHO NO LONGER PARTICIPATE IN MANAGED CARE

Litigation is only one way to resist. Perhaps the strongest and the bravest in the wounded profession of medicine are those doctors who seek to become insurance-free. They leave the paperwork to their patients, with the exception of patients who are covered by Medicare. Patients pay up front and submit their bills to payers themselves, in the old-fashioned way. Usually primary care providers—general practitioners or internists—these small-time rebels focus on patient care rather than administrative matters.

Two Washington, D.C., doctors who have sought freedom from administration have also sought freedom from the capitation system or the heavily discounted payment system that plans impose on participating physicians. With payment of about ten or eleven dollars per patient per month in HMOs in that region that work under capitation, Drs. Chretien and Corson figured out that they would have to see forty patients a day to earn $100,000 a year, a low-end salary for doctors working full time (Borbely, 2001: HE01). Actual discretionary income may be a very small percentage of that earned income. Most young physicians have medical-school debt to deal with as well as living expenses.

Per capita payment, it has been discovered via health services research, may not benefit the managed care plan. Many plans, by the way, are edging away from capitation because they want to make sure that participating physicians do not stint on service to patients. Still, highly discounted fees mean paperwork in order to collect from the plan.

Putting the onus on the patient to collect involves higher co-payments. What this rebellion of the docs means for patients are higher out-of-pocket costs. Not every patient will tolerate this new burden. Some patients leave, whereas others remain loyal to a physician whose work they respect. To keep patients, some primary care physicians keep their undiscounted fees at the same level as they were a decade or more ago. With fewer forms to fill out for the myriad of plans, doctors can spend less on overhead, that is, the cost of hiring billing clerks. With reimbursement by insurers up to the patient, doctors can focus on medical care *and* say "no" to the managed care steamroller. What this represents is

96   WOUNDED PROFESSION

individual, not organized, resistance in an age when organizations are
seen as the best defense against further erosions of the power and status
of the medical profession.

REFERENCES

Angell, M. 1993. "The doctor as double agent." *Kennedy Institute of Ethics Journal*
    3 (3): 279–86.
Bodenheimer, T., and Casalino, L. 1999. "Executives in white coats—The work
    and the world view of managed-care medical directors: First of two parts."
    New England Journal of Medicine 341 (25) (December 16): 1945–48.
Borbely, M. 2001. "This may hurt: some doctors are spurning managed care,
    giving more time—and a bigger bill—to their patients." *Washington Post*
    (October 30): HE01.
Center for Studying Health System Change. 1999. *Independent No More: How Ef-
    fective Have Physician Organizations Been in Responding to Managed Care?*
    Washington, DC: Center for Studying Health System Change (January 27).
    Available online at http://www.hschange.com/physconf/Transcript.
    html.
Emanuel, E.J., and Dubler, N.N. 1995. "Preserving the physician-patient relation-
    ship in the era of managed care." *Journal of the American Medical Association*
    273 (3): 323–29.
Freudenheim, M. 1995. "Doctors, on Offensive, Form H.M.O.'s." *New York Times*
    (April 7): D1, D7.
Gray, B. 1997. "Trust and trustworthy care in the managed care era: Can man-
    aged care organizations take on the mantle of trust that traditionally be-
    longed to physicians?" *Health Affairs 16* (1) (January/February): 34–49.
Hall, M.A., and Berenson, R.A. 1998. "Ethical practice in managed care: A dose
    of realism." *Annals of Internal Medicine 128* (March 1): 395–402.
Hilzenrath, D.S. 1998. "For doctors, managed care's cost controls pose moral
    dilemma." *Washington Post* (March 15): H01.
Kassirer, J.P. 1998. "Doctor discontent." *New England Journal of Medicine 339* (21)
    (November 20): 1543–44.
Kilborn, P.T. 1997. "Doctors organize to fight corporate intrusion." *New York
    Times* (July 1): A12.
Luhrmann, T.M. 2000. *Of Two Minds: The Growing Disorder in American Psychiatry.*
    New York: Alfred A. Knopf.
Mahony, M.A. 2000. *Saving the Soul of Medicine.* San Francisco: Robert D. Reed
    Publishers.
National Healthcare Cost and Quality Association. 2001. "RICO." http://
    www.nhcqa.org/bulletin.html 3 (1) (April).
Relman, A.S. 2000. "The crisis of medical training in America. Why Johnny can't
    operate." *The New Republic* (October 2): 37–43.
Rothman, D.J. 2000. "Medical professionalism—Focusing on the real issues." *New
    England Journal of Medicine 342* (17) (April 27): 1283–86.
"We should call it profit care, not managed care." *New York Times* (February 10):
    F24.
Wynia, M.K., Latham, S R., Kao, A.C., Berg, J.W., and Emanuel, L.L. 1999. "Med-

ical professionalism in society." *New England Journal of Medicine* 341 (21) (November 18): 1611–16.

Zielbauer, P. 2001. "Doctors sue health plans over coverage: Connecticut joins suits challenging H.M.O.s." *New York Times* (February 15): B1, B8.

7

How Managed Care Is
Shaping Medical Practice

Can the medical profession regain control over its own destiny? We cannot be certain that it will regain its prestige, power, and privileges without a carefully organized and orchestrated campaign to win back at least part of the autonomy it once enjoyed. Nor is it clear that academic medical centers (AMCs) will continue to be supported on the social capital derived from a public service approach to health care. It is also not clear whether the profession and the leadership from AMCs can do this without taking advocacy positions on major issues in health care today: the large number of uninsured, the shortages in nursing, and the need for the improvement of the quality of health care. These changes require forging alliances with the public and purchasers. Realistically, sustaining important services such as hospitals requires new federal and state legislation and collateral appropriations to subsidize these nonprofit institutions.

The medical profession cannot retake all lost ground. Managed care has rung in strong changes for medical practitioners in the mature markets where it dominates, and it will shape things as they come. Extreme market penetration in our metropolitan regions has helped rearrange the private practice system, making certain areas of concentration more interesting than they once were and helping newcomers to medicine, mainly women, make a smooth transition to independent practice. There also has been a fascinating geographic self-sorting and selection among physicians. Those who cannot abide by the rules and regulations of managed care, or the reduction in autonomy and incomes, head to greener

Table 1

SELECTED CHARACTERISTICS	PERCENT OF PHYSICIANS	
PRACTICE SETTING	1996–97	1998–99
Solo / 2 physicians	41%	38%***
Small group (3–10 physicians)	18	16***
Medium group (11–50 physicians)	6	7*
Large group (50+ physicians)	2.9	3.5*
Staff / Group HMO	5	5
Hospital owned	9	11***
Medical school	7	8
Other	10	12***
OWNERSHIP OF PRACTICE		
Owner	62	57
Not an owner	38	43***
PERCENT OF PRACTICE REVENUE FROM MANAGED CARE		
None	6	5
1–20	26	22***
21–40	28	28
41–60	19	21**
61–84	14	15*
85+	8	9***

Note: Statistically significant change from 1996–97 to 1998–99 at: *p < .05; **p < .01; ***p < .001.

Source: HSC Community Tracking Study Physician Survey, 1996–97 and 1998–99.

pastures where physicians can get better contracts or even practice without participation in health maintenance organizations (HMOs) or other managed care organizations (MCOs).

The trend in practice is toward joining large-group settings with fifty or more physicians, or hospital-owned practices. Increasing also is the percentage of physicians in medium-size or medical-school-sponsored practices. In contrast, the percentage of physicians in solo practice is declining, along with those in small group practices. Ownership of the practice has gone from 62 percent in 1996–97 to 57 percent in 1998–99. The percent of the practice revenue derived from managed care has also increased during this time period (See Table 1 for more precise contrasts) (Reed, Cunningham, and Stoddard, 2001: 4).

At an earlier time, the salaried doctor was considered a failure. A licensed physician gave orders and did not take them. Working for a salary meant that you could not cut it as an independent practitioner in the fee-for-service world. In 1983, only 24 percent of all physicians were employees. Fast-forward to 1997, when 43 percent of all doctors in practice were employees (Bodenheimer, 1999: 588). The captains of health care were no longer running the ship.

Health care planners suggest, as mentioned in earlier chapters, that the United States has too many doctors, particularly too many specialists. The Council on Graduate Medical Education (COGME, 1996) calls for better balance between the two types of practitioners as well as a reduction in some locations of physician supply to 145–85 clinically active physicians for every 100,000 people. Current estimates are that there are between 195 and 200 doctors for every 100,000 people in the United States.

This oversupply in American medicine has often been cited as producing too much unnecessary service when specialists are readily available. Since managed care, particularly the kind dispensed through the HMO model, is built around primary care and prevention, careers in this area of concentration have been receiving more financial compensation than in the past. Although it has often been viewed as a gratifying practice, primary care was not perceived by the profession as particularly attractive. The hours were long and the financial rewards were not commensurate with the time devoted to keeping people well. And primary care doctors were "on call," meaning they had to be available at night and on weekends to respond to their hospitalized patients. In contrast, subspecialties were seen as being at the frontier of new knowledge and applications as well as being involved in life-saving activities. Extra training and the responsibility of dealing with life-threatening situations were seen as justifications for additional remuneration for services rendered. The acute-care model dictated the rates of payment both by what the insurers and the patient paid out-of-pocket.

At its best, managed care attempts to keep people well. Even when patients suffer from serious chronic illnesses, the emphasis is on disease management and maintaining the person within her family environment. When bearing the financial risk, managed care providers seek to keep the patient out of the hospital and thus attempt to offset costs of hospitalization with the use of community-based care. Even when a person is hospitalized, modern practice, with or without managed care, initiates the patient discharge planning process twenty-four hours after admission. New roles are created for physicians as hospitalists: doctors who manage to safely shorten a patient's length of stay after admission through advice to the admitting doctor and assistance in orchestrating care.

The kinds of safeguards to keep a patient from lingering longer than necessary may be extremely important with managed care shaping medical practice. One strategic analysis of a national study found that patients with chronic diseases who are insured in prepaid managed care systems have 15 percent fewer hospitalizations than expected for individuals with the same medical conditions with different insurance coverage. Using data from 1986 to 1990 from the Medical Outcomes Study, 1,681 older patients with hypertension, diabetes, heart attack, or congestive heart failure were tracked longitudinally in three cities in the practices of 367 clinicians. Eugene C. Nelson, Colleen A. McHorney, Willard G. Manning, and others (1998) compared hospitalizations, office visits, and insurance payments for managed care and fee-for-service patients. No attempts were made to determine whether lower rates of hospitalization were related to good clinical outcomes, general health status, and satisfaction with care.

The decision by benefits officers at America's corporations to go with managed care has made it difficult to replicate this study in the twenty-first century. A research design that compared managed care with indemnity coverage might be a thing of the past. It should be pointed out that this kind of study could only be done using a Medicare or Medicaid population since traditional fee-for-service coverage is rare in today's insurance market.

Once the decision to hospitalize a patient is made, to what extent do managed care doctors seek out less expensive alternatives—avoiding or reducing the use of the intensive care unit (ICU)—compared with those doctors who are less cost conscious? Choosing the less expensive alternative would seem to fit right in to the cost-conscious style of managed care medicine. The ICU costs anywhere from three to five times the per diem rate for a regular inpatient bed. A study of 1992 hospital discharge summaries from Florida and Massachusetts found that extreme demand for placement in the ICU was a better predictor of length of stay than whether patients were in HMOs. Yet Bernard Friedman and Claudia Steiner (1999) found that even when the ICU bed census was down, HMO and self-paying patients had shorter stays than those with traditional hospital insurance, independent of the patients' clinical features. The ongoing reduction in hospital bed units in the United States, as the growth of managed care relentlessly reduces the need for excess capacity, should make for shorter stays as well as fewer admissions, regardless of the form of payment.

It is often noted that managed care medicine is significantly less reliant on specialty care. Using several techniques to discourage referral to specialists, MCOs impose financial penalties on patients who go outside the network. They also offer greater revenue to primary care physicians (PCPs) when they retain patients. Refraining from making referrals leads to the acquisition of payment withholds that serve as bonuses for PCPs who send patients to specialists within the limits set in advance for a medical group practice. Finally, physicians who know that patients in certain plans will suffer substantial out-of-pocket expenses if they go outside the plan are less likely to make those referrals (Grembowski, Cook, Patrick, and Roussel 1998).

Managed care has also made physicians more conscious of not prescribing incorrectly or ineffectively. National surveys of medical directors and primary care physicians conducted by Project HOPE's Center for Health Affairs found that

HMOS use four tools to affect PCPs' prescribing of pharmaceuticals: 1) the establishment of a drug formulary or the list of recommended or required drugs; 2) encouraging PCPs to prescribe generic drugs; 3) tracking individual PCPs' drug-prescribing rates and 4) educating PCPs about drug-prescribing. (Mueller, 1998)

The use of the formulary was far and away the most common technique used by managed care organizations to keep prescription costs down, followed by encouraging PCPs to prescribe generic drugs.

Although clearly incremental reforms, all these techniques ratchet down resource utilization. This should make the cost of care in the United States less expensive than in the past. The reliance of MCOs on primary care is a significant departure from the way American medicine is practiced. Specialists hospitalize more frequently than generalists. Specialists order more tests than generalists. With this information in hand, managed care organizations prefer to contract with primary care physicians such as internists rather than with subspecialists within internal medicine, for example, gastroenterologists. Fewer opportunities to see patients means less income for specialists, some of whom have decided to become generalists.

This trend should pick up as fewer specialists are required in the future. What factors or characteristics of the specialists encourage changing to primary care? Do all medical specialties yield to the new market trends at the same rate? Some specialty practitioners are more likely than others to change to general practice. According to University of Pennsylvania researchers, who examined practice changes among 335,000 physicians from 1982 to 1986, specialists who entered primary care fields tended to be female, graduates of foreign medical schools, and in hospital-based practices. In particular, subspecialty internists and pediatricians, emergency medicine physicians, and pathologists were more likely to change than doctors in other specialty practices. Many of those who changed practices already were viewing general medicine as a secondary emphasis in their practices. Physicians most comfortable with general practice while still specialists might be most easily recruited to primary care practices (Christakis, Jacobs, and Messikomer, 1994).

Today's physicians are very different from their counterparts who practiced during the golden age of fee-for-service medicine. Doctors, unhappy with their financial arrangement or organizational constraints imposed by MCOs, may not only join new plans but change their geographic locations more frequently than a decade ago. There are now doctors who serve as headhunters for disgruntled doctors seeking greener pastures. From the early 1990s on, 10 percent of the physician workforce changed jobs, whereas before that decade, less than 2 percent relocated. Perhaps free agency, as in major-league baseball, is the next step, making the scramble for jobs even more interesting.

The commercialization of health care, and particularly the way medicine is practiced, has not gone unnoticed by members of the profession. There are many incentives to get with the program, and many doctors now take business courses while in practice. Those most resigned to this change have joined the ranks of physician managers, who see the new mobility of doctors as something doctors have to anticipate and not grieve over. Howard Horowitz, M.D., vice president of the American College of Physician Executives, bluntly makes the case that times have changed. In an interview with a science reporter from the *New York Times*, he takes a position that more professionally oriented physicians, such as Arnold Relman, would regard as heresy.

As I see it today, the business of medicine is first a business . . . Today's health care industry is framed around power forces such as corporate integration, cost cutting, mergers and acquisitions, and attempts to reduce the number of health providers at less successful managed care organizations. As good as a clinician a particular doctors may be, sometimes the circumstances of the marketplace gang up on him. (Markel, 2001)

There is definitely a new way of thinking about the practice of medicine. Gone are the days when physicians were known as "Doc" and simply hung their shingle and waited for patients.

Dealing effectively with changing circumstances under these conditions rather than living well may be the best revenge. Aspiring doctors understand this as well as the most nimble of corporate executives. Consequently, the interest of medical students in becoming primary care physicians has increased as opportunities for specialty care have diminished. Incomes for family physicians, pediatricians, and other generalists have increased in the past decade, making these fields more appealing to young doctors than in the past. With medical school debt a burdensome responsibility, knowing that one will be able to pay it off steadily is reassuring.

Help is also available from professional associations that give advice on how to deal with managed care plans. Additional support is available from federal sources, including the Maternal and Child Health Bureau, a branch of the Health Resources and Services Administration (HRSA), an agency that is part of the United States Public Health Service that provides technical assistance to physicians or agencies struggling with packaging and setting fees for services, entering and participating in the managed care market, securing a contract with a managed care organization, negotiating a financially sound managed care contract, and obtaining adequate reimbursement for the services a physician provides. Experts on managed care at the HRSA Technical Information Center assist in all facets of contract negotiation. Free or low-cost services are available by phone, at the doctor's workplace, or through workshops that teach staff about managed care and appropriate reimbursements.

And there is more than merely cursory help. Individuals with senior-level experience review proposed and existing contracts and provide a written analysis. This analysis includes discussion of the adequacy of payment, risk arrangements, termination clauses, and enrollment procedures. Recommendations and suggestions for modifications of contracts are included, with on-site assistance available in contract negotiations.

It would be interesting to know how many doctors or organizations take advantage of this service. Managed care has certainly created a market for various intermediary services in the health care industry. Some of these organizations have been less successful than the "dot.gone" companies of the year 2000. Physician practice firms, once the darlings of Wall Street, have declared bankruptcy, and various hospital/physician partnerships have risen and split back into their original pieces.

The purchaser-driven marketplace for doctors has produced more changes than health care planners. Seeking to rationalize the health care system could accomplish more thorough changes than through policy initiatives alone. Clearly some bad days are ahead for specialists if current trends continue. To reduce sharply the numbers of physicians in practice would require reductions in the number of places in medical schools and internships and residencies in academic health centers and community hospitals, as well as limit the licensing in the United States of foreign medical school graduates. Some residencies would have to be restricted to reduce the excess number of specialists entering practice.

Not all of these conditions are brand new. Geography and demography have always played a big role in determining where physicians practice after their postgraduate training. Some areas were looked down upon because chances of generating an income sufficient to pay back student loans and also live an upper-middle-class lifestyle were slim. In the past (and still today), physicians avoided rural areas, such as the

Upper Peninsula of Michigan or the state of Maine, leaving health care in those regions in the hands of osteopaths and chiropractors. Today, labor-force-style research suggests that the presence of HMOs has made some metropolitan regions inhospitable to specialists. Specialty practice is highly dependent on referrals. The high market penetration of MCOs has led to fewer specialists, after training and fellowships, setting up their practices in those MCO-dominated metropolitan areas. And more of them are now relocating from those areas to friendlier regions (Escarce et al., 2000). The rates of increase in specialists is curtailed by the increasing presence of MCOs in a given area. Although still rising, the number of specialists in the United States is calculated as increasing at a slower rate compared with the past.

Not all changes are market driven, but they may still work to the advantage of the managed care world. The changing gender balance in medicine also has had an effect on the ratio of generalists to specialists, one that fits comfortably with the MCO model of service delivery. The growing percentage of women medical school graduates has also slowed the growth of the numbers in specialized medicine. Women are more likely than men to enter primary care residencies such as pediatrics or family medicine. Also, they are more likely than men to hold salaried positions and to work less than full time (McMurray et al., 2000). Attitude surveys suggest that female, compared with male physicians, are more likely to be concerned with balancing professional and family responsibilities. A large organization can offer flextime,whereas a specialist in solo practice may not get to know his children or walk his dog.

Some change is coming in the kinds of organizations in which physicians practice. And group practice fits in better with desires to balance professional and family responsibilities because there is someone to provide "backup" on a regular basis. Nevertheless, some organizational styles remain in place. There is evidence to suggest that the older ways of practicing are slowly changing though not completely gone. Even in the state of California with the longtime presence of the large group or staff model HMO—Kaiser-Permanente—many more specialists are found in solo practice (41%) compared with generalists (34%) (Dower et al., 2001: 28).

Being in solo practice does not prevent physicians from joining networks called independent practice associations (IPA). These organizations create the provider capacity that sells the managed care plan to benefits officers at corporations that purchase health care coverage for their workforce. IPAs not only negotiate with the MCOs on behalf of the physicians, but perform various administrative functions as well. In some states, again with California in the lead, 90 percent of generalists in urban areas belong to at least one IPA. Specialists tend to participate less, with only 54 percent in the Golden State involved in IPAs (Dower et al., 2001: 32). Because these doctors constitute a "virtual" partner-ship—most of the participants have never met—doctors can maintain their solo practices and work with other physicians.

Surely it must be an unusual experience to refer patients to complete strangers or accept referrals from complete strangers. Despite the large number of physicians who are solo practitioners, there are established networks among doctors who have learned over the years to trust each other. They have also learned to informally boycott physicians who have acquired a reputation for not practicing in an optimal fashion, irritating their colleagues, or exercising poor relations with patients. It is not con-sidered smart to maintain a well-developed professional relationship with someone who is universally avoided, even shunned, because of poor doctoring.

One of the benefits of creating these new networks of doctors, how-ever, is the opportunity to learn from others and avoid becoming "the doctors who are avoided" by practicing medicine badly. Nancy Keating and her associates, in their Massachusetts survey of more than 750 doc-tors, found that those who were in group practices or HMOs rather than solo practices were in hospital-based or community-center practices rather than private offices, and that those who received some income from capitation were more likely to use informal consultation. Primary care physicians were more likely to use these conversations than spe-cialists, with the opportunity to gain advice perceived as a way to gather information about how to better serve patients (Keating, Zaslavsky, and Ayanian, 1998).

Despite this reassuring set of findings, the existence of doctor networks does not mean networking is frequent, nor can patients be sure their doctors actually consult each other. To offset the discomfort associated with working among a strange panel of doctors, a screening process of physicians takes place. Most MCOs require that doctors permitted to work for them be credentialed. This review of qualifications—a kind of minimalist board certification—has been used as an accelerated but func-tional equivalent of building trust informally. Physicians not invited back to renew their contracts with MCOs may be rejected because of their lack of competency as physicians, or because they are inefficient users of scarce and expensive resources. They make too many referrals, perform too many tests, or too often decide in favor of the most expensive alter-native, such as surgery.

Watchful waiting, always among the least expensive treatment op-tions, has become more and more popular as managed care gets estab-lished. The old medical style of decisive intervention has not held up well under the onslaught of managed care. Whereas the salaried doctor may do just as well being thoughtful rather than action oriented, the modern day, newly minted specialist may still find it necessary to treat rather than wait. The old medical maxim, "If you don't treat you don't cure," may take on new meaning, one with a dollar sign on it, when smaller numbers of patients are passing into your examining room. At the same time, a physician who delivers unnecessary care today is more likely to be discovered than in the past. The use of computerized records to track physician practice behavior would make it very difficult to err on the side of surgery to remove a healthy organ.

THE QUEST FOR QUALITY AND EFFICIENT USE OF RESOURCES

Sometimes quality and cost savings are mutually supportive objectives in health care delivery. Hospital-based computerized record keeping made it possible to determine whether duplication of tests was occurring at a hospital in Massachusetts. Bates, Boyle, and Rittenberg (1998) found that 28 percent of twelve standard laboratory tests were redundant, occurring within test-specific intervals. Repetition of tests could be justified if the symptoms persisted, following the first test with results within normal limits. Yet there was no clinical indication for 92 percent of the repeated tests following results that showed normal results. The authors suggested that using computerized reminder systems might eliminate unnecessary and expensive tests.

Health services research has also benefited from the kinds of data that are now being collected systematically on clinical practices. The use of data on the delivery of health services has focused the spotlight on the inappropriate practices of primary care physicians (PCPs). Although they may be economical when it comes to testing and referral, PCPs endanger the public health of the nation via the overuse of antibiotics. Moreover, some of these treatments are ineffective as well as expensive. Mark Chassin, an expert on the quality of care (1998), reported that in 1992, 21 percent of all ambulatory antibiotics were administered inappropriately to treat colds, urinary tract infections, and bronchitis—all viral infections that do not respond to antibiotics. Alternatively, four known effective treatments for heart attacks were used on only about half the eligible patients. Because more than 750,000 Americans suffer a heart attack each year, proper use could lead to a reduction of about 18,000 preventable deaths (Chassin, 1998). The health care services industry, despite its life and death nature, tolerates more errors per million events than is found in most American industries. Quality improvement is within our reach but requires recognition that changes are in order.

New technology is augmented by new approaches to disseminating information about medical interventions that can make for more effective treatments. Evidence-based analyses seek to inform health care providers of more effective combinations of treatment modalities. This is most readily evident in a project funded by the Agency for Health Care Policy and Research and the National Institute of Mental Health—a five-year scientific study of how to improve outcomes in the treatment of schizophrenia. This project, part of the Patient Outcomes Research Team (PORT) series, is aimed at improving the quality of care for several high prevalence and expensive to treat diseases.

Central to improving outcomes in the treatment of this devastating mental illness was the adoption of a strategy that uses correct doses of appropriate medications and patient and family education and support. More refractory cases required aggressive community treatment. The researchers examined the extent to which patients with this brain disorder were receiving this effective treatment. They found that fewer than half the patients under treatment received the right doses of antipsychotic medications and psychosocial interventions (Lehman, 1998).

PHYSICIANS' VIEW OF THE QUALITY OF CARE

One of the medical profession's most interesting efforts to respond to the inroads managed care has made on medical practice has been to pick up the flag and lead the charge for improving the quality of care. Doctors who have spoken out on the issue of quality have generally accepted that in the struggle with managed care organizations, the profession of medicine will triumph if the public and the purchasers of health plan services believe the profession is on their side.

Although physicians in many countries perceive the quality of care as declining, the judgments of American doctors is that it is declining in unique ways (Blendon et al., 2001). American medicine is taking the lead in recognizing the need to improve quality in health care. In a Commonwealth Fund International Survey of specialists and primary care physicians conducted in five English-speaking countries in 2000, many physicians gave low assessments of the quality of hospital care. Respondents from the United States were more likely than those from other countries to point to interference with the way they practiced medicine and how this prevented their patients from access to quality care. Interestingly, very few American respondents said that there was a shortage of specialists or that waiting time was intolerable for patients who required special tests or procedures. The rationing of care found and so acutely felt in other countries, particularly Canada and the United Kingdom, was not a source of complaint in the United States.

In other areas under review American physicians' concerns were no different from those found in the other samples. Reducing medical error in hospitals was seen universally as a key goal. Forty-one percent of the 528 doctors in the United States survey said that they were not encouraged to report medical errors or that they were discouraged from doing so. Other problems with hospitals had to do with limitations on hospital care, with 38 percent of the American sample agreeing that they faced restrictions in admissions and allowing patients sufficient healing time before discharge. They also were more likely than doctors in other countries to object to the external reviews of their work and decisions by third-party payers.

Medical practice in the American sample was also hampered by formulary limits on drugs that could be prescribed (41%) and the high cost of prescription drugs (48%). This question of affordability is almost unique to the United States and New Zealand, and was not regarded as a major problem by doctors in Australia, Canada, or the United Kingdom. Again, in New Zealand (54%) and the United States (52%), physicians were concerned about out-of-pocket costs to patients.

Almost three-fourths of the physicians in every country were concerned about not having enough time to spend with patients. The burden of having to see many patients during the day, either to maintain revenues or because of contractual arrangements with payers, was lamented throughout the profession. In the land of the stars and stripes, however, 67 percent of respondents were concerned about the quality of care after hospitalization and 78 percent thought that better preventive services and patient education was needed.

In sum, American doctors were more likely than doctors in the other samples to think the entire health care system needed rebuilding. A higher percentage of doctors in the United States took this position than lay respondents.

Health services researchers have linked organizational and financial changes in American medicine to doctors' dissatisfaction with the practice of medicine, their thinking they have less freedom to care for patients in ways that are optimal, and their thinking their professional autonomy is restricted, because they perceive that managed care plans have moderate or strong incentives to shrink health service delivery A national study found that practicing good medicine is seen as difficult under these conditions. In 1997, Georgetown University health services researcher Jack Hadley and his associates conducted a telephone survey of more than 1,500 physicians from seventy-five large metropolitan regions. Fifteen percent of the respondents felt a moderate or strong pressure via incentives to reduce services. Compared with others in the sample, those who felt an incentive to reduce services were 1.5 to 3.5 times more likely to be very dissatisfied with their practices. They were also more likely to say that their professional standards were being compromised. They were more likely than other sample members to say that they did not have sufficient time with patients, and that their ability to hospitalize them, order tests for them, and make referrals was subject to interference (Hadley, Mitchell, Sulmasy, and Bloche, 1999).

Although complaints abound among physicians in managed care plans, no concerns were expressed about one area related to quality. No physicians interviewed suggested that peer review was being compromised by MCOs and their business practices. Protecting patients from inept physicians is not on the agenda. Nor do MCOs use the existing national reporting mechanisms to maintain quality by eliminating practitioners with deficiencies in practice or ethical standards.

MANAGED CARE ORGANIZATIONS AND INEPT PHYSICIANS

Students of the profession marked the beginning of the end of professional autonomy in American medicine with the introduction of peer and utilization review and with the advent of Medicare as nonmeans-tested public insurance for the elderly.

In 1986, Congress passed and President Reagan signed into law an act that created the National Practitioner Data Bank. Designed to protect patients against incompetent or unethical physicians who moved to another state when they lost their license in one state, the law sought to bring to light physician behavior that was censured or disciplined. However, with the growth of managed care, few plans contribute information related to such sanctioning to the data bank.

A recent study by the inspector general of the Department of Health and Human Services found that in the last ten years, only 16 percent of HMOs and 40 percent of hospitals made reports, comprising only 715 adverse actions. It appears that MCOs do not want to take the time to make a detailed report and/or are fearful of being sued by doctors who are reported for ineptitude or misconduct. An understanding is usually reached between the plan and a doctor who has been found guilty of misconduct, making it possible for the physician to resign from the plan, and without a report filed with the National Practitioners Data Bank. Although HMOs and other plans are required by law to make such reports, they are rarely disciplined when they fail to comply. According to health reporter Robert Pear (2001), "H.M.O.s and hospitals cannot be sued for errors they investigate and properly report. But if they fail to report discipline involving those errors, the government may remove the legal protections, a penalty that is rarely invoked" (p. A12).

The protection of the American public from inadequate practitioners seems beyond the responsibilities of managed care plans, even when they argue that quality care is their major concern. As with their failure to support medical education and training as well as public health sys-

tems that promote the common good, managed care plans simply walk
away and claim it is not their department.

REFERENCES

Bates, D.W., Boyle, D.L., and Rittenberg, E. 1998. "What proportion of common
    diagnostic tests appear redundant?" *American Journal of Medicine 104*:
    361–68.
Blendon, R.J., Schoen, C., Donelan, K., Osborn, R., DesRoches, C.M., Scoles, K.,
    Davis, K., Binns, K., and Zapert, K. 2001. "Physicians' views on quality of
    care: A five-country comparison." *Health Affairs 20* (3) (May/June): 233–
    43.
Bodenheimer, T. 1999. "The American health care system: Physicians and the
    changing marketplace." *New England Journal of Medicine 340* (7) (February
    18): 584–88.
Chassin, M.R. 1998. "Is health care ready for six sigma quality?" *Milbank Quar-
    terly 76*: 565–91.
Christakis, A., Jacobs, J.A., and Messikomer, C.M. 1994. "Change in self-
    definition in a national sample of physicians." *Annals of Internal Medicine
    121* (9): 669–75.
Council on Graduate Medical Education. 1996. *Fourth Report: Patient Care Physi-
    cian Supply Requirements: Testing COGME Recommendations.* Rockville, MD:
    Council on Graduate Medical Education.
Dower, C., McRee, T., Grumbach, K., Briggance, B., Mutha, S., Coffman, J., Vran-
    izian, K., Bindman, A., and O'Neil, E.H. 2001. *The Practice of Medicine in
    California: A Profile of the Physician Workforce.* San Francisco: The Center for
    the Health Professions.
Escarce, J., Polsky, D., Wozniak, G., and Kletke, P. 2000. "HMO growth and the
    geographical redistribution of generalist and specialist physicians, 1987–
    1997." *Health Services Research 35* (4): 825–48.
Friedman, B., and Steiner, C. 1999. "Does managed care affect the supply and
    use of ICU services?" *Inquiry 36*: 68–77.
Grembowski, D.E., Cook, K., Patrick, D.L., and Roussel, A.E. 1998. "Managed
    care and physician referral." *Medical Care Research and Review 55* (1): 3–31.
Hadley, J., Mitchell, J.M., Sulmasy, D.P., and Bloche, M.G. 1999. "Perceived fi-
    nancial incentives, HMO market penetration, and physicians' practice
    styles and satisfaction." *Health Services Research 34* (1): 307–21.
Keating, N.L., Zaslavsky, A.M., and Ayanian, J.Z. 1998. "Physicians' experiences
    and beliefs regarding information consultation." *Journal of the American
    Medical Association 280* (100): 900–904.
Lehman, A.F. 1998. "Schizophrenia PORT findings." *Schizophrenia Bulletin 24* (1).
    20-32.
Markel, H. 2001. "Doctors now need well-honed skills in job hunting." *New York
    Times* (May 22): F5.
McMurray, J., Linzer, M., Konrad, T., Douglas, J., Shugerman, R., and Nelson,
    K. 2000. "The work lives of women physicians: Results from the Physician
    Work Life Study." *Journal of General Internal Medicine 15*: 372–80.
Mueller, C. 1998. "Beyond the Gatekeeper: How managed care organizations

affect the use of technology." *Health Care Financing and Organization: News and Progress* (November): 5–6.

Nelson, E.C., et al. 1998. "A longitudinal study of hospitalization rates for patients with chronic disease: Results from the Medical Outcomes Study." *Health Services Research* 32 (6): 750–58.

Pear, R. 2001. "Inept physicians are rarely listed as law requires: U.S. program undercut. Study finds lack of reporting by hospitals and H.M.O.s—Lawsuits are worry." *New York Times* (May 27): A1, A7.

Reed, M.C., Cunningham, P.J., and Stoddard, J.J. 2001. "Physicians pulling back from charity care." *Issue Brief Findings from the Center for Studying Health System Change* 42 (August): 1–4.

8

Hopes for Reform

A popular American story in magazines and newspapers concerns the personal plight of physicians. They have fallen from grace; their status as affluent members of the moneyed class in American society has been shaken. And now they have to worry about making ends meet, paying bills, keeping their payrolls down, and possibly, having to become a member of the salaried classes. The enormous autonomy and control of the workplace that went along with the rise of professional dominance in health care in the 1960s seems an imagining of the past rather than bona fide memories. The unimagined height to which the profession soared seems outside the grasp of most newly-licensed doctors. Today, more doctors are looking inside the profession for guidance, seeking to remake the image of medicine as a means of improving its authority as an American institution. The struggle with managed care organizations appears to the observer to be somewhat on hold as the profession seeks sources of cultural renewal. Can the resolve of organized American medicine match the force of managed care—finance capital seeking to penetrate the citadels where medical knowledge, applied and pure, is generated, and where doctors ply their craft? As I write this chapter, there is more individual distaste expressed than organized efforts to fight back.

   With shattered dreams comes new recognition among doctors that the hurting is widespread. Although few medical practitioners are moonlighting as bartenders, there is a strong sense of outrage. The trendy *New York* magazine's August 6, 2001, cover story wasn't about steamy sex in the sultry city but doctors' anger toward the insurance companies that converted to managed care, patients who undervalue the services they receive because their co-payments are less than fifteen dollars, and the benefits officers who saw their chance to rein in the costs of health care at the expense of "club med."

Similar stories have appeared throughout the nation. However, *New York* is an excellent place for this kind of story since the island of Manhattan, the epicenter of Gotham, boasts a disproportionate share of the medical profession in America, a unionized workforce in hospitals and medical centers, as well as some of the planet's highest rents for office space. While journalist Steven Fishman's article "Doctor Feelbad" is a treatise about the money (or lack of access to it), it also chronicles the decline of occupational status and power. We learn that downward mobility in the new millennium affects not only Internet marketers at bankrupt dot.com companies, but those with framed degrees on their walls as well. Despite the fact that doctors are not seeking unemployment compensation, there is a real sense of being downsized as a profession. Writers in the business sections of our daily newspapers say that Enron, a once nimble corporation, has done its last jig; the same may be said for professions. Doctors are still dancing, but they are not calling the tune.

With the medical profession experiencing collective anxiety, some popular analogies dealing with downward mobility spring to mind. Will Bruce Springsteen write rock anthems about belt tightening among professionals in the oughts ('00s) as he did about the loss of lunch pail industries and blue collar jobs in the 1980s? I don't think so. We will see a spate of cartoons on the subject in the *New Yorker*, a publication that reflects social changes, including downward mobility, with some subtlety.

Still, downgrading has some rewards. The American public finds the profession of medicine trustworthy and deserving of admiration. Yet one cannot help but feel that some of this support manifests itself in the form of sympathy for the vulnerable. Who knows how deep this support really is? World support for Israel is at its highest when it suffers military defeats at the hands of its Arab neighbors. Doctors may be in a similar situation when it comes to acquiring positive numbers in American public opinion polls—the numbers may reflect a bad situation but not indicate that medicine is being replaced by another profession on a faster track.

Clearly, this heavyweight contender has wounded pride. The Fishman article, and others like it, enable doctors to sing the blues, to say they are mad as heck and won't take it anymore. But these songs of financial woe are short on analysis and ways to make quality health care available for all at reasonable cost. And they leave out the remedies proffered by health policy gurus and the leaders of medicine to help this proud profession regain its cultural authority and social standing. Who are the leaders in this effort at reprofessionalization? What will it take to make American health care an institution that is more about quality and less about reining in costs?

The directive to look inward is no better expressed than in a "Piece of My Mind" column in the *Journal of the American Medical Association* (Hundert, 2001). What drew me to the article initially was the fact that the author had the same name as a college-age friend. The title, "A Golden Rule: Remember the Gift," didn't attract me as much as the author's name. Aside from the fact that the article was full of concern for patients, it also suggested that medicine might be a kind of sectarian group—one in which mutual respect among the membership produces respect from the outside. Hundert goes on to say that

the most important and unappreciated cause of the public opinion crisis about American medicine is the way in which attitudes of respect *for ourselves* (for better, or mostly for worse) get projected outward to the community. As the basic structures of medicine are being reshaped and people are questioning the very integrity of American medicine, I say it is time to look inward.

In seeking an inward-based renewal the medical profession may be a latecomer. The writings of Dr. Hundert sounded more than faintly familiar to me. More than twenty years ago I wrote a theoretical article on reprofessionalization in pharmacy, suggesting that the displacement the profession experienced via the end of compounding and the reduction of owner-operated community pharmacies led that profession to look inward (Birenbaum, 1982). As I observed in writing about pharmacy for better than a decade, there was a sense that it was becoming a social movement, not just a profession. A kind of jingoism prevailed among recent graduates of pharmacy schools that the profession was about to change the world, or so it seemed to those captured by its spirit of professionalism.

I looked for guidance on how to interpret what I saw within the scholarly literature that had enlightened me as a graduate student and practicing social scientist. It was exciting to find parallels in the literature on cultural change as a response to transformations in the social structure. Sociologists and anthropologists who studied religious transformations among various dispossessed peoples in the nineteenth and twentieth centuries designated these responses "revitalization movements." Wallace claims that revitalization movements always originate in situations of social and cultural stress and are in fact, an effort on the part of the stress-laden to construct systems of dogma, myth, and ritual which are internally coherent as well as true descriptions of a world system and which thus will serve as guides to efficient action (1966: 30).

Although Wallace was looking at contemporary societies, it should be noted that religious movements of the eighteenth century in Europe also responded to social change by seeking to create a new set of tenets to guide the brethren. And nineteenth-century America produced similar shock waves among the established churches and some sectarian movements that sought to keep the dynamic American society at arm's length.

At the time I wrote about the changes in pharmacy I saw medicine as being secure, with many other health professions in its shadow. Before the managed care revolution I would not have seen any use in characterizing this dominant profession as troubled. There is little doubt today that medicine is under stress as a profession at the same time that individual practitioners are, transparently, stressed. There is fear of downgrading and partial displacement by nurse practitioners and physician assistants in the area of primary care. More significantly, there is a shared fear of loss of control over scarce resources and loss of a capacity to deal with uncertainty according to clinical judgment acquired through training and taking charge of—that is, being accountable for—patient care. Furthermore, the forms of organizing medical practices, as was shown earlier, are not meshing well with the new realities of health-care financing.

Many physicians complain that the business end of medicine is sullying the patient care environment, making it difficult to communicate clearly with patients (Conigliaro, 2001). The business end has become central to practice, obscuring the core mission of practitioners.

At the core, medicine is about human encounters on a fundamental intimate level. The desire to form a close relationship to directly help another person has driven the practice of medicine throughout the ages. We now spend much of our time entangled in discussions of managed care contracts and cost effectiveness, all the while carrying out our duties to examine, diagnose, prescribe and operate. (Firlik, 2001)

The old relationships have become so fractured that health service researchers and policy analysts who study the regional differences in relationships between payers and providers focus a great deal on variability in market settings for providers to demonstrate that some autonomy is possible. The autonomy and control spoken of in these studies concerns avoidance of capitation and utilization review requirements, two features of managed care that doctors find odious. Most of these forms of freedom translate into resistance to cost reduction measures rather than struggles to be in charge. What it often comes down to is that when buyers of insurance squeeze the managed care companies, the squeeze is then applied to providers. To wit: The higher the average commercial health maintenance organization (HMO) monthly premium for single coverage, the more freedom from cost-cutting measures. Physician organizations are hardly a force for change under these tolerant conditions, even less so when they are in surplus and where purchasers of coverage are not very generous (Rosenthal, Landon, and Huskamp, 2001).

How did the old relationships between payer, provider, and patient unravel? How do the leaders of medicine seek to restore the original mission of medicine when payers are no longer willing to sustain professional autonomy and the traditional guild system that supported its cultural authority? What would be the best outcome for assuring the continued improvement of the quality of medical care and the elimination of the continuous inflation that has led to the payer rebellion? I will attempt to use each of these questions to bring to a close this treatise on managed care and the profession of medicine.

DISEQUILIBRIUM

The profession of medicine, to some extent, today is a victim of its success in limiting interference with its growth during its golden years. Although attempts were made to limit expenditures through the regulation of the health care industry during the 1970s and 1980s, little was done to prevent medical schools and residency programs from producing more doctors, particularly subspecialists, than are required to prevent illness, keep patients well, and treat sick people. The incentive system dictated professional behavior. The way doctors and hospitals gained remuneration in the service-intensity driven fee-for-service system was to do as much as possible. This formula for success discouraged the selection of the least expensive treatment options or the use of one's time as a provider to do modestly compensated preventive interventions.

The result was that many procedures were unnecessary and sometimes dangerous for the patient. Provider-induced demand went along with the practice style that was dominant in the profession. With the preferred focus on providing the kind of care that is rewarded by privilege, power, and prestige, newly minted doctors eschewed primary care and sought to do the dramatic interventions that went along with tertiary care. And because most graduates of medical school in the United States took out large loans to pay for their tuition, the best way to pay them back was to seek out a specialty that was well compensated.

The American health care system, spurred on by the need to continue and even increase physician incomes and expand the jurisdiction of medicine, was actually good at keeping people dependent on more and more service, but it was not very good at preventing people from getting to the point where they needed acute care in abundance. Additionally, the profession made few efforts to create universal coverage. Only the federal government had sufficient reach to create insurance for all. For U.S. physicians, the government was a menace. Physicians did not want the government to mandate health care to all, even when it would only increase their remuneration. Employer mandates for coverage during the halcyon days of health care reform were anathema to private practice doctors who paid their employees nonunion wages and provided few insurance benefits.

The health care system grew as the population aged and belief in technology prevailed. Doctors were up to their eyeballs in patients as Americans sought assistance in maintaining youthful lifestyles; getting things corrected while they were covered by Medicare or private insurance; and making frequent visits to be monitored, have medication changed, or petition for a prescription even when it was not indicated. It is difficult for physicians to say no, and it helps retain patients to say yes. It was only in the 1990s that limits were established in the name of cost-driven goals. The introduction of managed care forms of organization made it clear to decision makers that more care was not necessary. A health care recession followed briefly as the focus shifted from inpatient to outpatient care and procedures and from specialization to primary care.

The surplus capacity of the American health care system is clearly reflected in the disproportionate number of specialists to generalists along with thousands of unfilled beds in hospitals and medical centers. Moreover, when regulation made it harder to admit patients and keep them in hospitals, specialists found ways of providing their services on an outpatient basis. This situation often left doctors competing for patients with hospitals with which they were affiliated. By diverting patients so they could perform procedures in ambulatory care settings, hospitals were often the victims. Hospitals were already bleeding at the margins through the introduction of the prospective payment system via Medicare. Not long afterward, insurance companies introduced this payment system for their covered lives. The result was that as lengths of stay were decreasing, extra bed capacity was increasing. They became financially vulnerable and subsequently were willing to contract with payers in the form of managed care organizations to give deep discounts to these organizations to provide inpatient care in exchange for patients to fill their beds.

At the same time, by responding to financial pressures and incentives initiated by managed care organizations, doctors, as a guild, lost control over how they were paid. Dictating the fee structure was now out of their hands. A significant disequilibrium occurred when a critical mass of doctors willingly joined managed care plans. Now they would discount their fees, work under capitation, or become salaried in exchange for access to patients. When employers encouraged their employees to join HMOs or other managed care plans, they were asking patients to give up complete choice of their regular sources of care in exchange for savings, whether by avoiding deductibles, or paying lower co-payments and premiums. Consequently, benefits officers became convinced that their firms' funding for health care insurance would go further and be used more efficiently than in the past. In fact, despite a reduction in the use of the HMO model, most firms today offer one plan—take it or leave it.

The rapid progression to managed care forms of financing health care had, by 1998, left only 12 percent of the commercial insurance population under traditional indemnity coverage, wherein physicians were paid in an unaltered customary and prevailing fee-for-service system. Most doctors, if they were to maintain their incomes, had to enter into contracts with managed care organizations. What this also produced was an eclipse of professionalism, that is, dedication to patient well-being, or in a larger sense, a community orientation as opposed to an orientation to individualistic gain. As the philanthropist George Soros (1999) said in his inaugural remarks about the "Medicine as a Profession" project at his Open Society Institute,

Clinical care is now dominated by for-profit corporations that place the interests of the shareholders above the interests of patients and often disregard the ethical obligations of doctors. Health care companies are not in business to heal people or save lives; they provide health care to make profits. In effect, in the necessary effort to control health care costs through the market mechanism, power has shifted from physicians and patients to insurance companies and other purchasers of services. (p. 2)

LEADING REPROFESSIONALIZATION

The profession needs to reeducate itself and then reeducate consumers as to the virtues of voluntary simplicity as a way to limit unnecessary utilization. From the liberal perspective, the health care system uses up scarce resources that could be reclaimed to educate our children better, provide moderately-priced housing, or increase mass transportation. From the conservative perspective that free choice is sacred, it does not allow consumers command over how they want to manage their health care dollars or allow them to invest as they see fit. On the public side, from a conservative perspective, it also competes with funding for a (questionable) national missile shield. Most Americans would agree that domestic security is important, especially after the events of September 11, 2001. Whatever your alternative uses, there are ways to shrink health care to more manageable proportions as other countries do.

Medicine as a profession has not made a concerted effort to teach the public that there are priorities within the world of health care. In a country built around a strong belief that "what's in it for me" rules all priorities, this may be a hard sell. Still, there is good reason to believe that the public is educable. Consider how successful seat-belt laws have been in promoting compliance (and saving lives). For a long time, policy experts believed that only passive restraints made sense because they believed that Americans would not take to buckling up.

The same thing applies to other forms of learning, including recognition that there are times when heroic intervention is useless. Scarce resources in the intensive care unit cannot be effective for everyone. Doctors have learned how to teach patients' relatives and friends when to withdraw life supports. Medicine must be the guardian of medical resources because few other professions, public officials, or consumers have the knowledge to make choices about when to end the life of a person on a dying trajectory. These decisions have to be based on preserving the quality of life for patients and their families, not just for the sake of saying that everything was done or that the rules prevent us from going further in extending life. Health care proxy agreements and living wills also help us let go of the patient in end-of-life situations.

The need for lifestyle changes is also getting higher priority in medical practices. Primary care physicians in all HMOs that participate in the quality control and improvement programs sponsored by the National Committee on Quality Assurance are required to open discussion about smoking, its dangers, and smoking cessation programs. Although these are worthwhile activities, still more can be done to discover conditions that need to be treated, such as hearing loss, not just behaviors that lead to expensive care thirty years later.

More abstract, but equally important, are efforts to provide population-based health care, a form of prioritization whereby physicians in a particular area determine the health care needs of the community based on demographic and epidemiologic data. To treat asthma effectively, for example, doctors have to know where the highest risks for the disease reside in the community, not just treat the most easily accessible. Treatment also involves family education to help keep patients with asthma well and out of hospital care.

Consumers and patients would listen more closely to what doctors and health policy experts say about prioritizing the use of scarce resources if more respect and admiration were expressed for the profession. There is a strong need to institutionally retain the essence of why young people want to become physicians—to serve society and humankind. This altruism needs to be maintained throughout the careers of physicians and not be lost once medical school is completed and residencies acquired. Expressions of continued caring and compassion will generate respect for the advice the profession gives and will provide public legitimacy to the prioritization of medical needs.

Physicians need to volunteer their time and sit on community advisory boards, both related to health care services and the provision of other public goods. They need to hear directly from laypeople what their needs are. The sharp separation between the professional and the lay world needs to be eliminated as the representatives on both sides need to learn how the other half thinks and what it values. Critical thinking is not reserved only for those who attended medical school. There is much to be learned from patients and their families. Cultural diversity exists even within the same ethnic community when the worlds of the highly educated, the educated, and the less educated meet. There needs to be a dialogue between representatives of these different cultures.

NEW FORMS OF COLLECTIVE REPRESENTATION
FOR PHYSICIANS

The older associations—the county and state medical societies—that made it possible for doctors to control the price and distribution of medical care in the community, and their national organization, the American Medical Association, no longer represent the majority of physicians in the United States. The closed ranks of medicine found in the local societies, with threats of loss of malpractice insurance if one didn't belong, or loss of referrals from fellow doctors, failed to prevent the managed care revolution from happening.

Older doctors who could not work under the new forms of payment and control took early retirement or became medical examiners for life insurance companies. Even the latter were replaced by physician's assistants at half the price. Again, insurance companies were making their own rules and doctors were being priced out of the market. Some doctors advertised their services as expert witnesses, showing a willingness, for a substantial fee, to testify in medical malpractice cases. This further reduced the social solidarity of medicine. The profession still had its specialty associations, although their national and even international scope made it less likely that they could influence voters or legislators. And as we all well know, since politics is local, personal ties are needed to move decision makers.

Regaining complete control over the health care delivery system by the profession will never happen again, and it should not happen. We would be deceiving ourselves if we believed things were better in 1972 than they are in 2002. The gravy years of fee-for-service, with third-party payment, were times of overtreatment and an enormous waste of resources. Sometimes unnecessary services were downright dangerous for patients. Today, as consumers worry about undertreatment or stinting on services, we must be concerned about services being too little, or even too late. Keeping costs down is everybody's business, and doctors and patients can work within the same organization to promote efficiency as well as limited use of unnecessary treatments.

The profession of medicine needs to become imbued with a spirit of partnership, one that can help improve quality and increase access and delivery services at more modest costs. This willingness to partner with other constituent groups in the field of health care could be done if other groups acquired the same spirit. Working out a structure of cooperation through partnership means that neither government nor corporations gain the upper hand in controlling health care. A balance between government intervention and profit making has to occur so that the rights of patients and professionals are respected.

This approach has been designated a *civic community* model by Lois Wright Morton (2001). Much like the civil society imagined by the reformers who ended the necrotic rule of communism in Eastern Europe, it is based on socially constructed limits to state power through the development of intermediary organizations. It strenuously eschews rampant individualism, also know as libertarianism, a moral code that says there should be no restrictions on access to services or commodities so long as the buyer has control over choices. Believers in this kind of individualism celebrate capitalism and the power of the market to deliver what is needed to all. True believers in the superiority of the marketplace in health care ignore the success of Medicare and Medicaid in promoting access to life-extending services.

For Morton, the way to avoid the extremes of the one-size-fits-all approach and the unregulated market is to create mechanisms for control that increase involvement of the actual producers and consumers of health care. It is a form of cooperation in which those who must seek health care and those who deliver it have extensive input into the design of services as well as those who deliver the services. Payers and regulators have to respect this involvement.

[I]ndividuals of multiple organization design the institutions that respond to health care needs; social choices can be evaluated on more than a materialistic and monetary standard; economic actions are not separated from social morals and actions of society; and sustainability depends on the involvement and actions of individuals in the community. (p. 140)

The key example offered by Morton for how such a civic community can be accomplished is the development of the Oregon Health Plan, a scheme to increase access to health care for the near poor by reducing expenditures on big-ticket items that assisted only a few covered by Medicaid and/or were questionable in their effectiveness. The determination for how this would be done was through the development of an allocation system that was publicly created, explicit in its intent, derived from consensus, and accountable to the citizens of the state (Morton, 2001: 160). An eleven-member Health Services Commission (comprising five physicians, four consumers, a public health nurse, and a social service worker) was established to oversee the process. Health-care providers of all kinds, as well as constituencies that might be adversely affected by newly established priorities, were able to give testimony at commission hearings. Additional information and opinion was collected at community meetings and a telephone survey. The commission then ranked health services according to their comparative effectiveness and the population to be served.

With nearly all individuals below the federal poverty line covered by insurance, some key indicators of the public's health showed improvements. More pregnant women received prenatal care than in the past, and the infant mortality rate dropped significantly. Expensive procedures such as heart transplants were permitted under conditions where they were critically needed and where they would be most effective (Morton, 2001: 163).

Although this is an exciting example of partnering among many different types of consumers, such as people with disabilities, and providers (physicians and academic medical centers), the players did not include any health insurance companies, pharmaceutical manufacturers, or for-profit hospitals and nursing facility chains. We have yet to see the for-profit sector engage in the kind of exchange and compromise necessary to work out arrangements that all the players can live with. Government agencies, and the elected officials who run them, can participate more easily than corporate leaders in these kinds of social experiments since they are accountable to the electorate every four years. They are shielded for longer time periods than corporate leaders who have to respond directly to owners. The stockholders of Big Pharma will show their displeasure by selling off their stock, thereby reducing the value of the company, or by voting to eliminate offending corporate officers at annual meetings of all the owners.

Moreover, the "take-charge" culture of corporate America makes partnerships unlikely between players with differential amounts of power. Consequently, we need to consider how medicine can take the lead in connecting these disparate interests so we can move forward. We need to consider how it can provide better care and more productive use of labor, and help us withstand the kinds of shocks that the unforgettable year 2001 brought to our country.

REFERENCES

Birenbaum, A. 1982. "Reprofessionalization in pharmacy." *Social Science and Medicine 16*: 871—78.

Conigliaro, R.L. 2001. "Review of *Communicating with Today's Patient: Essentials to Save Time, Decrease Risk, and Increase Patient Compliance.*" *Journal of the American Medical Association 286* (6) (August 8): 725.

Firlik, A.D. 2001. "Review of *A Piece of My Mind: A New Collection of Essays From JAMA, The Journal of the American Medical Association.*" *Journal of the American Medical Association 286* (6) (August 8):

Hundert, E.M. 2001. "A golden rule: Remember the gift." *Journal of the American Medical Association 286* (6) (August 8):

Morton, L.W. 2001. *Health Care Restructuring: Market Theory vs. Civil Society.* Westport, CT: Auburn House.

Rosenthal, M.B., Landon, B.E., and Huskamp, H.A. 2001. "Managed care and market power: Physician organizations in four markets." *Health Affairs 20* (5) (September/October): 187—93.

Soros, G. 1999. "Medicine as a Profession." Available online at http://www.soros.org/medicine/gssspeech.htm (April 15), p. 2.

Wallace, A.F.C. 1966. *Religion: An Anthropologic View.* New York: Random House.

9

The Future of American Medicine

We have looked at the past and present situation of the medical profession in the United States. To end this treatise on managed care and the profession of medicine, I will first put the future of medicine into the context of the aftermath of September 11 and the recession of 2001. This connection is not merely pandering to the reading public or making the obligatory bow to the momentous event of the new millennium. I resisted introducing the infamous atrocities of that date in this book before now, until it occurred to me that it could be instructive. We need to consider the disruptions of health care security that many felt in New York, particularly in the financial district when jobs were lost. When lives were lost, the widowed also lost health care security in the form of insurance. Discontinuities in health care coverage rise to the surface when the economy goes into a steep decline. Where in the personal, yet political process of loss of employment-based health insurance and the unaffordable costs of insurance premiums for others can the profession make a difference? Can medicine preserve its autonomy and enhance its stature by being better advocates for consumers? Can the private troubles of doctors be made into a public issue?

The second task is to analyze the directions in which medicine as a profession is headed, given the trends propelling it toward increased dependence on technology for clinical practice and highly capitalized health care plans for income and access to patients. These changes at the workplace level require a personal and a political response. They are structural conditions that threaten to make clinical work less meaningful and more socially isolating, with less control, greater self-estrangement, and less opportunity for self-actualization. Readers familiar with the literature on the sociology of work and its nineteenth-century forerunners will recognize immediately the components of alienation. What can the profession do to prevent the reduction of professional autonomy? Are there ways for physicians to promote increased self-actualization and meaningfulness in the workplace?

POST-SEPTEMBER 11 AMERICAN SOCIETY

The United States had its domestic security and tranquility challenged when commercial airliners were converted into weapons of mass destruction on a beautiful, bright Tuesday morning on the East Coast. It is hard to feel safe in our usual haunts when almost 3,000 people died at their workplaces at the World Trade Center and the Pentagon. The psychological trauma has brought psychiatry and related fields to the forefront. Healing will be short- and long-term. The lives of children have been affected by the loss of parents and grandparents and by the enormous exposure on television of endless replays of the destruction of the World Trade Center towers. The United States has called upon psychiatrists, psychologists, social workers, and clergy to help us deal with grief and recover a degree of security in our daily lives. The efforts of health care providers who gave their time and wisdom will help improve the public image of the medical profession.

The profession has probably also regained some stature as a result of its willingness to deal with the long-term casualties of the suicide attacks in New York and Washington, D.C.

The United States may never be the innocent place it once was. Flying the friendly skies will no longer be operative. We are told to go back to our jobs and shop until we drop. At the same time, we are expected to be vigilant. Guardedness and lighthearted behavior don't mesh well. We turn to the professions for guidance in a darker world. The mysteries of Islamic fundamentalism need some explaining. In turn, the mysteries of direct or indirect trauma require interventions by mental health experts; and, notwithstanding mental health service being available, participation in communal actions is required to make us feel like we are part of something larger than ourselves.

Even more status-enhancing has been the response of public health experts, including clinicians, to the bioterrorism, from whatever source, that was generated by the letters mailed to the United States Senate and some media headquarters. In the future, we will need to be prepared to respond to continuations of the distribution of highly-refined anthrax and, inevitably, copycat kinds of attacks. Perhaps the American public will have a greater appreciation for those in the health care field who do not perform dramatic interventions the way thoracic and neurosurgeons do, but who are vital in eliminating disease such as yellow fever and malaria through public health measures.

Despite gains in prestige, the profession has not regained the power lost to managed care in the financing, organization, and delivery of health services. Physicians in the United States are finding their incomes and control over their work situations in decline. This is occurring, ironically, without the introduction of "socialized" medicine, a term used to refer to doctors becoming paid state employees or dependent on the government financing of health care. State-controlled medicine is often viewed as rule-ridden and painful for physicians. Can it be that different from working in an HMO, a private bureaucracy?

As I write, there is very little concern in the United States with state-controlled medicine and a great deal of concern with managed care in the for-profit sector, making life difficult for physicians. Market forces are clearly powerful factors in reversing the fortunes of the profession. Doctors now compete more directly for patients than at any time since states began seriously to license the profession. And the profession has become more and more dependent on health plans to gain access to patients.

The squeeze on medical providers has happened without health care reform. Fear of government intervention led to a rejection of universal coverage and guaranteed access to health care for all. Many doctors opposed the employer mandate, as it became known in 1994, because they didn't want to provide coverage for their employees. With the reduction in the number of doctors in solo practice and small group practices, there may be an opportunity to revisit health care reform. Fewer doctors want to keep their expenses down in small private practices today.

Advocates for a single-payer system, as found in Canada, argue that when there is only one payer, the providers are in a difficult bargaining position and have to keep their charges down. Over the past decade, even with a considerable number of payers, U.S. doctors have provided deep discounts to insurers, both private and public, to get and hold on to patients. Medicaid and now Medicare, as payers, have demanded and received a discounted fee structure. The community-based rate—referred to as customary, prevailing, and reasonable—is rarely paid, except perhaps by affluent individuals who seek out doctors who don't accept insurance. Within the profession, there is much talk but little effort to regain the power and prestige lost in the era of managed care. Revisiting the past, for a profession on the decline, becomes a comforting way to take control of the future.

Some look back to that golden age of American medicine when doctoring permitted professional dominance and insurers did not dictate how medicine was to be practiced to guide the future. Life was much more pleasant when medical men, and I choose this gender deliberately, did not have to deal with rules and regulations created by private and public payers. Professional dominance is like any other kind of extreme mastery in the work place. There was an Eden-like quality to it. Hegemony makes power holders think that this is the way it always was and that this is the way it always will be. The disavowal of wrongdoing in the profession by its leadership was extraordinary. The professional standards in American medicine during the 1950s were self-serving. And to be sure, not all the financial practices engaged in before the advent of managed care were ethical. Much in the way of unseemly behavior on the part of doctors is swept under the rug when old-timers yearn for a return to the epoch before Medicare and Medicaid. To paraphrase Eugene McCarthy, the liberal anti-Vietnam war senator from Minnesota, when commenting on the demeanor of Ronald Reagan, they imagine the past and remember the future.

The social historian David Rothman (2001) reminds us that the golden age was replete with behaviors and values we would find unacceptable today.

Fee-splitting was pervasive, and so was conflict of interest (through physician ownership of small hospitals and dispensing of drugs and equipment); medicine was an upper-middle-class, white male profession, with a marked antipathy for women and minorities. Organized medicine was fiercely anti-governmental, working hard to subvert national health insurance. And, as others have remarked, it may have been a great day to be a doctor, but it was a lousy time to be a very sick patient. (p. 2605)

The concern that medical spending was uncontrolled, a perception that propelled corporate benefits officers to seek managed care contracts with health maintenance organizations (HMOs), has been modified slightly by the enormous prosperity of the Clinton years. Despite the fact that not everyone shared in the surpluses produced during these boom times, the consensus was that we were getting our economy in order and that our national government was becoming more fiscally responsible. Companies, consumers, and the overseers of Medicare and Medicaid were pleased that the rate of increase of health care costs was decreasing. The federal deficit and the national debt were being paid off, and it was time to give tax refunds and loosen the restraints a bit in other ways. But neither the American leadership nor the public were prepared to deal with the atrocities of September 11, 2001, and the U.S. economy was not prepared to deal with the fallout that followed.

CHANGING MANAGED CARE AND THE FIRST
RECESSION OF THE NEW MILLENNIUM

Although the economic march of the longest growth period in our history may have ended in March 2001, the official start of the recession, the day of the attacks on New York and Washington, DC, and the failed third attempt, ending in a crash in rural Pennsylvania, remains the symbolic start date of the new challenge to the United States. Better preparation for the unexpected—war and a recession—might have occurred had President George W. Bush not been so smitten by the idea of giving tax breaks to the wealthy. Imagine how federal surpluses could promote military mobilization without borrowing, assist states in paying for the burdensome costs of special education or Medicaid, or keep Social Security safe from cuts or increases in payroll taxes to meet the demands of the baby boomers.

It can be said that before the current recession, managed care was a-changing. We may see a reversal of fortune as freer choice of providers becomes more widespread. In recessional times, these changes, including the movement to expand patient choice may end before we know it. Still, it is useful to review what has been given back to beneficiaries, especially since physicians find these changes salutary as well. It has not all come from employers seeking to placate employees. Physicians who engage in "pushback" have been somewhat successful in reducing their financial risks, gaining leverage through consolidation, and creating bigger provider pools for health plan members to choose from (Draper et al., 2002: 16).

During the unparalleled expansionary period that lasted nearly ten years, managed care made rapid advances in the insurance industry and among self-insured corporations, but a scarcity of labor, combined with impressive profit making, led employers to soften some of the stricter and disliked aspects of their medical benefits plans. A striking parallel was the largess of employers during World War II when they introduced hospital insurance to reward workers and hold on to them during a period of wage and price controls because medical benefits were outside the confines of inflation fighting by the government.

Let's take a closer look at what has happened and not happened. Many of the predictions of the past decade about the end of fee-for-service medicine in America and the triumph of the capitation system have proven wrong. The fastest-growing sector of managed care is called the preferred provider organization, or PPO, and it has prospered by reducing restrictions on patients and their doctors. Even a number of the more highly organized HMOs have reduced the requirements to see primary care providers before seeking help from subspecialists (Selis, 2001). It is getting harder and harder to tell the difference between PPOs and

HMOs, according to some of the benefits experts. "Frankly, all these plans are starting to look alike," says Paul Fronstin, director of the health-research program at the Employee Benefit Research Institute in Washington, D.C. "Anyone trying to describe the differences is just going to confuse things" (Selis, 2001: 24).

Today, many employer-sponsored managed care plans do not require primary care physicians to serve as "gatekeepers" to specialists. Authorizations for procedures are also viewed as coming forth more quickly in PPOs than in HMOs. Medicaid and Medicare HMOs still operate with the primary care physician as the key coordinator of care. Doctors find it more professionally appropriate when they are able to get their patient referrals completed without interference from external reviewers.

Another retreat for managed care came in the public insurance sector. Medicare HMOs are now few and far between, as health plans respond to new restrictions on their federal financing that has made them less profitable than in the 1990s. Physicians may rejoice that fee-for-service Medicare will remain the predominant way in which senior citizens gain access to medical care. What has also hurt HMOs in the Medicare market has been the extraordinary increase in the cost of prescription drugs. As pharmacy benefits are cut back at HMOs, Medicare recipients with heavy expenses for prescription items no longer find these health plans attractive (Freudenheim, 2002: C1).

Increasing costs may return us quickly to the barracks capitalism of the HMO. The triumph of this consumer-oriented health care system comes with major costs. Managed care contracts for the year 2001 rose 11 percent, increases that exceed inflation two or three times. Future annual increases are expected to be even greater. Facing rapidly rising premiums, benefits officers are now off-loading costs onto employees in the form of higher deductibles and co-payments (Freudenheim, 2001: C6). Patients are not only being asked to pay larger co-payments and deductibles than in the past, and are increasingly responsible for larger shares of the cost of prescription drugs, but they are also expected to pay a greater share of the cost of prosthetics.

At the same time plan enrollees are expected to shoulder more of the financial burden across the board, benefits managers are considering ways to squeeze savings out of the biggest users of health care plans—sick people. Employers are seriously considering shifting costs to individuals with several thousand dollars in medical expenses, whereas those workers who remain healthy or are not heavy users of health-care services will receive a bonus credit they could use against future medical expenses.

Built around a medical or health savings account, this kind of coverage is used to pay initially the full costs of hospitalization, prescriptions, or medical procedures. Once this account is spent, the enrollee pays out-of-pocket until an upper limit of spending is reached. At that point, coverage under the health care plan is triggered. Usually, this is accompanied by co-payments until another threshold is met, and then the plan covers fully any additional medical expenses.

Such a medical expense plan puts the burden of deciding *when* to get an expensive procedure done on the consumer. A person in need of a hernia operation, for example, may put it off to a future date when their medical expense account is refreshed with new contributions from the employer (Freudenheim, 2001: C6). Although such a procedure is elective, concerns may be raised by the medical profession when the unwillingness to spend because a medical expense account is exhausted or the treatment has to be paid for fully out-of-pocket clouds the judgment of someone in need of bypass surgery or another complex, expensive, but necessary procedure.

With a reduction in the share of health insurance paid for by employers, one can also imagine some agonizing scenarios. We may be returning to what life was like in the 1950s very soon, an era in which the elderly lived lives of quiet desperation. Before Medicare, senior citizens on fixed incomes had to make choices between purchasing food or medical services. The rates of doctor visits before Medicare were far lower among the elderly than they are today. Today, because of programs such as Medicare, the elderly are far healthier than they were thirty-five years ago.

Americans without health insurance today limit physician visits because they simply cannot afford them or because it might mean taking money away from other necessary expenses, such as food or shelter. The same situation may start to apply to the insured as well. Medical expense plans today may force an enrollee to choose between mortgage payments and an expensive medical procedure. Are benefits officers who find these kinds of medical saving account plans appealing suggesting that they believe less is more? Does insecurity make for a more careful sick person, one who wisely husbands his or her limited resources?

A similar kind of stress on the American public is being produced by the increasing costs of prescription drugs. Pharmaceutical products have become a major part of the Americans' lives. Not only is the drug industry a major business but it has had an effect on life expectancy. For those patients on limited budgets and multiple medications, expenses are often so burdensome that the choice between paying for prescriptions and food or shelter may not seem so outlandish, despite their having coverage.

At the end of the nineteenth century, impressive gains in life expectancy and the quality of life were the result of improvements in sanitation, pure drinking water, greater access to calories, and the introduction of personal hygiene practices, such as washing one's hands after using the toilet. Today, great improvements have been made in life expectancy because of immunizations, antibiotics, easier access to medical care (prevention, early detection), technological advancements (magnetic resonance imaging, brain scanning), and organ donation programs. Technology in health care, when it is decisive, as with the use of immunizations or antibiotics, usually saves lives and reduces the use of other health-care resources. However, the introduction of new procedures during the past twenty years has generated few offsets in cost. Technology can replace labor only in a limited way in health care: There is still a need for skilled and well-educated people to deliver medical care, operate MRI units, and harvest organs.

Better living through chemistry, the development of effective pharmaceutical and biotechnical products, also contributes to people living longer. The medical management of chronic illness, owing to the use of prescription drugs, is much more effective than in the past. These improvements come with a price—in 1999, 44 percent of the rise in health-care costs for the entire American population was caused by increases in the cost of prescriptions.

Longevity also means the need for more direct care staff, such as aides, companions, and home visiting, which leads to a discussion of how Medicare has changed since 1965. The model used then was Blue Cross and Blue Shield and commercial insurance coverage. There was little emphasis on prevention; health maintenance through medications to treat chronic illness did not exist. As a result, the Medicare program passed in the 1960s does not match the needs of the older population today. Planners of Medicare based the benefits package on what catastrophic illness costs were in 1965 and what kinds of treatments worked then. Clearly, back then, hospital care, in the form of per diem expenditures and medical care in hospitals, made up the biggest part of health care spending. Prescription medications were not a concern because the weapons available were limited and seniors paid little for medications. Few older people in the 1960s took as many as five medications a day, as many do now, and this does not even consider the increased use of vitamins and dietary supplements to prevent deterioration.

In the twenty-first century it is not unusual for eighty-year-olds to take a variety of prescription medications every day, medications they will continue to take for the rest of their lives. Prescribing, monitoring, and managing the drug interactions of several medications at the same time becomes a central task for primary care physicians with a high proportion of older patients. How this complex task can be accomplished within the confines of managed care, as well as other considerations related to being the patient's advocate, has produced interesting realignments among payers and providers.

Releasing primary care doctors from the task of husbanding resources has encouraged them to be greater patient advocates than in the recent past. James C. Robinson (2001), in writing about the end of managed care, regards this as the right role for physicians. The emphasis on financial risk assumption for medical groups contracting with health plans is receding because health plans are less likely to contract with groups than with individual doctors.

The natural role of the physician is as the agent of the patient, offering information, advice, service, and support. Physicians want to advocate for more social resources to be devoted to health care, not for balancing of their individual patients' needs with the other economic priorities of the nation. (p. 2627)

This noble statement is supported by a study done by Robinson and his colleague Lawrence P. Casalino that compares the scope of capitation contracting and delegation of responsibility for payment and medical management in New York and California. Using data obtained from Aetna U.S. Health Care and six provider organizations in the two states, the authors compared physician organizations and found a reduction in global and shared risk capitation (Robinson and Casalino, 2001). Health plans are finding it more and more difficult to work with large physician organizations, preferring to contract with individual physicians and to retain control over such tasks as network development, provider payment, claims processing, and medical management. Alternatively, as evidenced through some highly publicized lawsuits, a number of California physician organizations are claiming that the plans they have worked with have underreported information about their covered lives so they can pay less on a per capita basis. Rate setting has to be based on accurate information about utilization and the population being covered by insurance.

Something even more important may be heading our way when it comes to understanding where the profession of medicine is going. The force of health care reform—the quest for universal coverage and the right of access to health care—may be seen throughout the land once again. A recession often catches people anticipating income that does not come forth. Layoffs of substantial parts of the workforce are part of a strategy for firms to ride out a recession. Those laid off face direct problems, and medical debt is one of them. It has been noted that approximately half of all families that went bankrupt in the United States in 2001 cited an inability to pay expensive medical bills. Robin Toner, a *New York Times* news analyst, suggests that matters related to access to care and the high cost of insurance are once again on the national agenda. Policy makers face a dangerous blend of recession and soaring costs, and ordinary people are letting us know that life without insurance is scary (2001: A34).

A Commonwealth Fund telephone survey, conducted by the Princeton

Survey Research Associates in the spring and summer of 2001 with a random national sample of 3,508 adults, found that being without health insurance even for a brief time could have long-term health and economic ramifications for families. According to Karen Davis, president of the Commonwealth Fund, as quoted in an Internet report, "A lapse of insurance coverage, whether due to losing a job or inability to pay a premium, is strongly linked to lack of access to medical care, problems paying medical bills and even paying for basic living costs such as food or rent" (Commonwealth Fund, 2001). As far as financial consequences:

Half of uninsured adults and 44 percent of those with a time uninsured in the past year had problems paying medical bills.

One-fourth of the currently uninsured and 31 percent with any time uninsured in the past year had to change their way of life to pay medical bills.

Those who were fully or partly uninsured have difficulty paying for basic living costs such as food, rent, and heating or electric bills.

Additionally, respondents reported that access to health care was reduced because they lacked insurance coverage fully or partially during the year.

52 percent reported that they experienced one or more of the following access problems:

43 percent who were uninsured at the time of the survey and 31 percent of those insured now but uninsured for part of the year indicated they did not see a doctor when sick.

About one-third of all respondents whose coverage was affected did not fill a prescription or skipped medical tests or treatment.

One-fourth with no or partial coverage did not go to a specialist when referred.

In contrast, one in five of the fully insured reported one or more of these access problems.

Once again, Americans are beginning to feel insecure about their health care coverage. The last health care reform movement, starting around 1991, was also related to a recession in the United States. The surprising gubernatorial election in Pennsylvania in November 1991 is a case study of how much dissatisfaction with unmanageable medical bills led to the defeat of a well-known candidate with a huge and apparently insurmountable lead in the polls when the contest began.

In October 1991, Harris Wofford, a little-known Democratic candidate for Senate from Pennsylvania, narrowed the gap in his race with former Governor (and former U.S. Attorney General) Dick Thornburgh, by calling for national health insurance. The Republican candidate was caught without a position on what had become a vital issue in his home state. The 1980s were not kind to the Keystone State—it lost 400,000 well-paid manufacturing jobs, which were replaced with 500,000 service-sector positions. Unemployment was close to 7 percent. Workers and their families were losing benefits as well, and medical bills began to pile up.

The populist brand of politics, attributed to the advice of James Carville, was clear in the Democratic candidate's statement—"If criminals have a right to a lawyer, I think working Americans have a right to a doctor." Worried about medical bills and access to care, Wofford's message reached the middle classes of this former heavyweight industrial powerhouse commonwealth: starting 47 percentage points behind his powerful and prestigious rival, the labor-supported dark horse candidate won comfortably by 11 points.

As we enter a new recessional period, the immediate dislocation of 79,000 workers from Lower Manhattan, the result of the destruction of the World Trade Center, and surrounding neighborhood, provides graphic evidence of the need for universal coverage by a single payer. Health coverage equals security. Coverage should be in place, regardless of what catastrophes occur. If government-sponsored health-care insurance had been available to workers outside of their employers, either through New York State or a federally-sponsored program, workers and their families would not have had to scramble to become enrolled in Medicaid in fall 2001.

Who knows whether the dislocation of these largely service industry workers had an effect on the nonbinding referendum that passed in the state of Maine in November 2001? This reawakening of interest in universal coverage, to be provided by state government, passed by a 52 to 48 percent margin.

The insurance companies are taking this support for a government-based program very seriously. Anthem Blue Cross Blue Shield contributed $382,000 to a "turf roots" organization called Citizens for Sensible Health Care Choices to produce television advertisements, similar to the "Harry and Louise" commercials sponsored by the insurance industry and mentioned earlier in this report, that sowed doubt about the value of the Clinton health plan (Belluck, 2001). Similarly, we need to wonder whether the Democratic victories in gubernatorial elections in New Jersey and Virginia may have been propelled by the voters' fear of falling produced by a major national recession.

The ingredients for health care reform redux are there. Perhaps this time, the profession will lead the way to greater coverage.

COMEBACK

Where does the medical profession fit into this ever-changing environment in the health care arena? Will it help the profession if it works to put health care, once again, on the national agenda? Will the historical splits in the profession reemerge as they did during the abortive health care reform years in the early 1990s?

The profession views itself as a group made up of thousands of advocates for individual patients. As a player in the health care reform struggle, this self-image could manifest itself by taking positions that promote universal coverage and an end to the piecemeal system of insurance we have today in the United States. Leadership for this kind of effort will likely come from those in the profession who have lost the most in the conversion to managed care—the academic medical centers (AMCs) and the specialists affiliated with them. It was precisely this interest group, perceived as source of entrenched costs that were kept out of the discussion on health-care reform led by Hillary Clinton in 1993 and 1994.

A second source of support will come from physicians who have had to give substantial discounts on their fees to gain access to covered lives. As a result, they must see more patients each day to compensate for the reduced fees they receive. This group overlaps somewhat with the specialists at the academic medical centers, yet in terms of numbers, they may be found affiliated more with community hospitals than AMCs.

All these groups within American medicine have a stake in improving the quality of care, a stake that comes from an innate sense that this is the right thing to do. Managed care should not mean stinting on services, or organized underutilization. Life-threatening conditions need to be identified and treated, when an effective treatment is available, regardless of restraints from the payment system. The profession also will benefit when professionalism promotes high standards of service.

One of the most important services the profession can perform now is to communicate to the American public, lawmakers, and employers that continuity of care is not just an ideal but a necessity when providing quality care. The discontinuities in care suffered by employees who lost their health insurance, or, like many of the restaurant workers in Lower Manhattan, who never had it in the first place, should be obvious from the Commonwealth Fund survey summarized earlier in this chapter.

A second commitment is to make it clear to the insurance industry that medical necessity involves not only applications and treatments to help a person recover, but interventions to maintain functioning and prevent declines in functioning and the quality of life. An acute-care-oriented profession does not pay enough attention to the need for intervention when chronic disease and disability may be threatening a patient's well-being.

The profession of medicine needs to lead the fight to reduce the cost of medications under patent protection so that people with moderate incomes can afford to purchase them. Discounts should be available. In addition, the American public should not have to shoulder alone the burden of research expenditures in the development of new drugs. Other advanced industrial nations enjoy deep discounts from drug manufacturers, and their citizens should bear part of the costs involved in pharmaceutical product development. The medical profession cannot do quality work and help patients if drugs remain unaffordable to a large percentage of Americans. An impersonal, rather indifferent market should be tamed when it does not work for the majority in areas of life and death.

The enormous growth of medical technology over the past twenty years requires greater control over its use by the medical profession. A focus on quality should be a major concern of the profession, particularly at a time when the overuse, misuse, and under use of medical technology and its role in generating medical errors can be reduced (Chassin and Galvin, 1998). Excessive cost to consumers should also be a concern of the profession. Yet the belief that managed-care penetration may lead to stinting is something that experts on quality consider an issue for the profession. "Professionalism (i.e., putting patients' needs first)," writes Barbara J. McNeil (2001: 1617), an expert on quality improvement in medicine, "is an important factor that should encourage physicians to resist financial pressures to withhold necessary technology in providing care for a patient."

Although resistance begins at the point of contact with patients, there needs to be recognition within the profession that withholding appropriate interventions because they are expensive is not the same as withholding technology that results in only marginal improvements in patients. The profession, as an interest group, needs to back up physicians who stand up to pressures to keep expenditures down in managed care organizations (MCOs). Physician organizations should be actively involved in designing a health care system that increases access to care and improves substandard care (McNeil, 2001: 1618). It needs to convince the chieftains of the managed care organizations that this is a major task of medicine.

In sum, a generalized concern in the profession for quality will help promote the retention of control over clinical autonomy and advocacy for patients, the bedrock of professional autonomy. If the battle over professional autonomy is won, other strategies for standing up to MCOs, such as collective bargaining representation, may lose their appeal.

Some physicians see collective bargaining as helping to sustain clinical autonomy and to preserve and enhance the quality of care. Currently, approximately 27 percent of all clinical-care physicians who are past their training (residents and fellows) and are not public employees are salaried employees. Recognizing this shift to salaried employment, the American Medical Association, after many years of resistance, established a new organization, Physicians for Responsible Negotiation, which may become a bargaining agent for employed physicians.

Collective bargaining, a right protected under the National Labor Relations Act (NLRA), excludes supervisory employees. When the National Labor Relations Board recently tried to extend collective bargaining protections to supervisory nurses, their argument was rejected by the Supreme Court, based on the fact that nurses, by exercising independent judgment at work, are subject to the supervisory exclusion clause of the NLRA (Choudhry and Brennan, 2001: 1141–42).

Currently, no consensus exists in medicine on the value of the trade union approach to dealing with management. The American Medical Association has supported collective bargaining for physicians and, as I write, is lobbying for amendments to the NLRA that will limit the supervisory exclusions. Some physicians believe collective bargaining will lead physicians to limit their control over their work, even involving walking away from their professional responsibility to optimize care for patients. Choudhry and Brennan (2001) assert the following:

In our view the provisions in labor law that prevent unionization by physicians are appropriate from the viewpoint of medicine as a profession. Physicians in practice do act independently, and those who are employed frequently manage and supervise clinical care. Physicians need to be able to manage and supervise in order to carry out their professional responsibilities. Clinical autonomy and advocacy for patients require the kinds of activities that members of bargaining units cannot participate in. (p. 1142)

Organizing efforts by physicians who are independent contractors and seek to bargain collectively runs afoul of existing anti-trust laws. To do so would be considered price-fixing, since one contractor is supposed to be competing against every other contractor. There is a middle way, however. The Department of Justice and the Federal Trade Commission in 1996 issued a statement that gave the go-ahead to physicians who wished to create networks for joint ventures. Calling them "safety zones," the statement said that if members of a network shared financial risk and did not constitute more than 20 to 30 percent of all physicians in particular practice in a specific geographic area, they would *not* be subject to anti-trust enforcement by the legally responsible agencies.

Whatever road is followed by the profession—unionization or independent contracting—there will be no quick or painless reduction to its alienation. Even well-paid work can have its discontents. Some in the profession will call for new forms of organization to produce social change. This is inevitable as the profession continues to remain silent in the face of a growing reduction in access to health care owing to more Americans losing employer-based health care insurance as they become unemployed. The profession also has not come up with a strategy to deal with the vexing problem of how doctors are to maintain their roles as friend, confidant, and significant service provider to their patients. Although the prosperity of the nineties led to a loosening of managed care restrictions to help hold on to valued employees, current members of the medical profession may be faced with belt-tightening measures. Few physicians can survive without joining managed care plans. Yet joining may mean implementing cost-cutting measures that might endanger the lives and well-being of patients. How members of the medical profession deal with the inherent role conflict produced by participation in MCOs will be a closely followed issue in this decade. Whether the profession forms a partnership with consumers will also be an important indicator of health security in our nation.

Professions, which start out as altruistic and knowledge-based occupations, seek to control their own fate. Autonomy in their control and practice always requires that the profession give something back to society. The medical profession in the United States, for the good of the public, should be leading the charge for health care reform, not just reacting to what payers dictate. And the charge has to be undertaken. All Americans require health insurance to promote the use of appropriate care, create more equal access, and get everyone to take some financial responsibility for their health care. No commercial insurer can price their product low enough for low-income families to be able to afford coverage. Industries that are made up of companies that do not provide group insurance need targeted interventions to promote group coverage.

Health care has become a business, made up of commercial enterprises that watch the bottom line. Despite the concern about costs, there seem to be few remedies. There is a cry from the public for relief from having to pay a great deal for insurance and prescription drugs. What is happening with the elderly and prescription drugs is the tip of a nasty iceberg that creates stress for other age groups, although not as keenly felt as with senior citizens. Whether the U.S. medical profession will engage in a partnership to extend health benefits to all, promote quality care, and still avoid increases in national expenditures through the performance of unnecessary procedures depends on the profession's realization that autonomy and control have to be there to promote the commonweal and not to navigate according to the profit motive.

REFERENCES

Belluck, P. 2001. "Small vote for universal care is seen as carrying a lot of weight." *New York Times* (November 16). Available online at wysiwyg:// 6//http:www.nytimes.com.
Chassin, M.R., and Galvin, R.W.1998. "National roundtable on health care qual-

ity. The urgent need to improve health care quality: Institute of Medicine National Roundtable on Health Care Quality." *Journal of the American Medical Association 280*: 1000–1005.

Choudhry, S., and Brennan, T.A. 2001. "Collective bargaining by physicians—labor law, antitrust law, and organized medicine." *New England Journal of Medicine 345* (October 11): 1141–44.

Commonwealth Fund. 2001. News Release: Loss of Health Insurance Jeopardizes Health and Economic Security of One in Four Working-Age Americans (December 12). Available online at www.cmwf.org.

Draper, D.A., Hurley, R.E., Lesser, C.S., and Strunk, B.C. 2002. "The changing face of managed care." *Health Affairs 21* (January/February): 11–23.

Freudenheim, M. 2001. "Employees are shouldering more of health care tab: Survey also finds costs rose 11% in 2001." *New York Times* (December 10): C6.

———. 2002. "Many Medicaid Plus Choice plans dropping prescription drug benefits." *New York Times* (January 25): D1, D6.

McNeil, B.J. 2001. "Shattuck lecture—Hidden barriers to improvement in the quality of care." *New England Journal of Medicine 345* (November 29): 1612–19.

Robinson, J.C. 20001. "The end of managed care." *Journal of the American Medical Association 285* (May 23/30): 2622–28.

Robinson, J.C., and Casalino, L.P. 2001. "Re-evaluation of capitation contracting in New York and California." *Health Affairs—Web Exclusive*, W11–19.

Rothman, D.J. 2001. "US Medicine," a review of *Severed Trust: Why American Medicine Hasn't Been Fixed*, by George Lundberg, 2000. *Journal of the American Medical Association 286* (November 28): 2604–05.

Selis, S. 2001. "The PPO identity crisis." *Health Leaders: Information to Lead 4* (December): 24–27.

Toner, R. 2001. "A stubborn fight revived: Parties dig in on the matter of health care and insurance." *New York Times* (December 20): A34.

Index

About the Author

ARNOLD BIRENBAUM is Professor in the Pediatrics Department of the Albert Einstein College of Medicine and Associate Director of the Rose F. Kennedy University Center for Excellence in Developmental Disability Education, Research, and Service.